New 800 Calorie HCG Diet

Richard L. Lipman M.D.

Biography

Richard L. Lipman M.D. is a board-certified internist and endocrinologist in Miami Fl who has treated more than 30,000 individuals with weight and metabolic disorders. A graduate of the University of Pittsburgh, he did his internal medicine training at the Universities of Pittsburgh and Miami. Dr. Lipman was Assistant Chief of Endocrinology at the USAF Hospital in San Antonio, Texas while in the Air Force, during which time he authored 18 publications in metabolism. To date, he has published 10 books on metabolism and weight loss.

Content

Introduction

Imagine a weight loss program that involves no surgery or starving, no outrageous exercise program, no dangerous pills and no expensive prepackaged foods. Imagine a diet that satisfies all your cravings, allows you go to restaurants and won't leave you feeling tired, hungry, or irritable. A diet like this been available since 1954! It's the HCG Diet invented by the British physician Dr. A.T.W. Simeons. This 500 calories a day HCG Diet has helped overweight men and women decrease their appetites, increase their metabolism and quickly lose inches from their hips, thighs, stomachs, and buttocks. Dr. Simeons' HCG diet combines small doses of the hormone Human Chorionic Gonadotropin (HCG) with a 500 calories a day almost zero carb food plan. Dieters reshaped their body and lost up to 1 lb a day. Dr. Simeons' findings were published in his 1954 booklet **Pounds and Inches** which can be viewed at BestBuyHCG.com.

There has been much criticism of Dr. Simeons' HCG diet since its publication in 1954 despite millions of people around the world experiencing often profound weight loss. The severity of the calorie reduction to only 500 calories a day and the almost complete elimination of almost all carbohydrates are only part of the problem. Furthermore, the Simeon' plan also restricts exercise, cosmetics, and personal hygiene products and requires daily injections of HCG hormones. All of these requirements have made it difficult and too burdensome in today's fast-paced world.

Miami internist and endocrinologist, Richard Lipman M.D. has treated more than 3000 patients with his new, improved HCG plan. Dr. Lipman's HCG Plan is a modern weight loss program that integrates the basics of the original HCG diet with results from current medical studies to provide a system that has been clinically shown to rapidly burn fat while maintaining lean muscle mass and protecting from protein deficiency. It is a medically based program built around an 800 calorie a day, low carb diet coupled with small doses of HCG that is simple, easy to follow whether one has 10 or 100 lbs. to lose.

What You Will Find in Dr. Lipman's Plan:

- Board Certified Internist and Endocrinologist treating HCG patients for 12 years.
- HCG resets your hypothalamus reducing hunger and re-setting metabolism.
- Easy: No injections, the strongest, purest HCG drops under the tongue! No killer workouts no special foods.
- Effective: Lose ½ to 1 pound per day!
- Lasting: All the secrets to speed up your metabolism permanently (Phase 3).

How is Dr. Lipman's Plan Different?

- Dr. Lipman is an endocrinologist like Dr. Simeon. He has updated all the new information since Dr. Simeon wrote his original diet in 1954.
- Updated food plan using hundreds of new, low calorie, no sugar, no fat foods. Based on high protein at each meal, prevents hunger, feelings of deprivation and ensures variety.
- "2 + 4" rule for selecting foods from a food label.

How Can You Eat Only 800 Calories a Day and Not Be Hungry?

- The food has minimal carbs which reduce hunger. At the same time is high in protein.
- HCG drops reduce hunger.
- Fat mobilization with HCG and mild ketosis produced by the diet lowers hunger.

More About HCG and Fat Burning

The word "hormone" causes one to think in the sex sphere. Other natural chemicals like thyroid, insulin, cortisone, adrenalin are also hormones that are not related to any sexual function. HCG is a hormone produced by the uterus only during pregnancy. It serves as a back- up a system to nourish the growing fetus even if the mother lacks sufficient caloric intake. It is produced in enormous quantities, so that during certain phases of pregnancy a woman may excrete as much as one million units per day in her urine (by comparison, in this plan you might be taking less than 500 units a day). HCG is not a sex hormone.

HCG never makes women look like men nor does it feminize a man. It neither makes men grow breasts nor does it interfere with their sex function. "Gonadotropin" usually means a "sex-related" hormone; however, no amount of HCG is ever able to increase normal sex function.

The HCG hormone also speeds up the metabolism, by signaling the body to burn more fat. HCG products can safely be used by both males and females who need to lose weight. Following the HCG diet protocol, your metabolism will operate over 30% more efficient to burn stored fat. HCG opens only the surplus fat cells allowing excess fat to be burned. This does not happen at other times in the human body. Other diets often remove fat cells that the body needs. HCG forces you to burn the excess fat cells eliminating the unneeded fat. You will be literally sculpting the body and losing inches as well as pounds.

Dr. Simeons described three distinct kinds of fat. He wrote that "two fats we need, and one we don't." If you've tried dieting and found that the weight comes back, it's because diets can't burn the one kind of fat that most needs to be eliminated - abdominal fat. Here is how Dr. Simeons described storage of body fat.

Three Different Fats in the Human Body

1.) **Structural Fat** is the first type of fat. It fills the gaps between various organs and acts as a protective barrier. Dr. Simeons describes this fat: "Structural fat also performs such important functions as bedding the kidneys in soft elastic tissue, protecting the coronary arteries, and keeping the skin smooth and taut. It also provides the springy cushion of hard fat under the bones of the feet, without which we would be unable to walk."

2.) **Reserve Fat** is the second type of fat which fuels the body when the nutritional intake is insufficient to meet the body's needs. Normal reserves are localized all over the body.

3.) **Abnormal Fat** is the third type of fat which has the potential of providing fuel for the body, but rather than being available for nutritional emergencies, it is locked away in fixed deposits. Often just below the skin of the abdomen and buttocks, it is the visible fat that people want most to eliminate. We have recently learned that there is another fat not fully recognized by Dr. Simeons that is stored inside the abdomen around various organs that is the most important of all fat deposits. This fat, called visceral fat produces chemicals that can travel through the bloodstream. These chemicals can raise blood pressure, cause cancer, raise cholesterol, interfere with insulin function, and even cause polycystic ovaries and infertility.

An MRI of an obese and thin man below illustrates the different types of fat deposits:

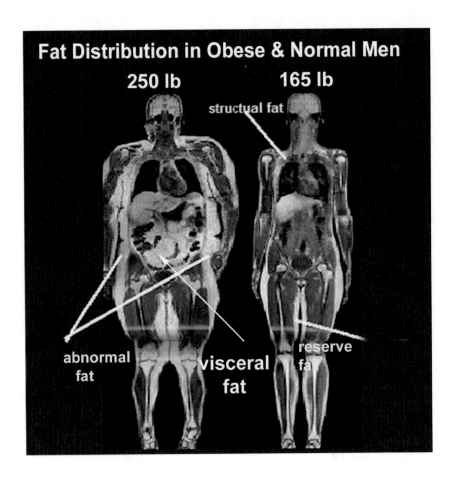

How Fat is Mobilized

In studying various weight loss programs, Dr. Simeons found that when patients starved themselves, they first lost their Reserve Fat, and after that, the Structural Fat. In the HCG plan, the "abnormal fat" is mobilized first. That's the fat that most people want to eliminate. Dr. Simeons explains these fats and weight loss: "When an obese patient tries to reduce by starving himself, he will first lose his normal fat reserves. When these are exhausted he begins to burn up structural fat, and only as a last resort will the body yield its abnormal reserves, though by that time the patient usually feels so weak and hungry."

Other Clinical Uses for HCG

HCG is clinically used both to induce ovulation and treat certain ovarian disorders in women. HCG is utilized to stimulate the testes in hypogonadal men (men who are not producing testosterone.

Updating the HCG Diet for the 21st Century

HCG Diet has been used by millions of dieters around the world over the past 65 years. No organized diet plan to my knowledge has been used so safely by so many people for so long of a time. Most of the research on the diet dates from 1950's thru early 1970's and is mostly patient weight loss results. Some studies found enhanced weight loss with HCG while others have revealed no differences. Most research studies have shown less hunger with HCG and some studies found muscle preservation and more fat loss after the HCG diet. Asher and colleagues reported in Clinical Nutrition in 1973 a 19 lb weight loss over 6 weeks in patients treated with HCG injections compared with an 11 lb weight loss in placebo-treated patients. All followed the same 500-550 calorie carb restricted diet using the Simeons protocol.

A small study by the American Society of Bariatric Physicians (now called the Obesity Medicine Association) published in the Bariatrician in 2012 revealed a 30% increase weight loss with HCG vs. those on conventional weight loss diet. Dr. Sheri Emma MD. reported on the Dr. Oz show in 2012 that HCG dieters lost 21/2 times more fat than muscle. Her report of over 1000 patients demonstrated the safety and effectiveness of the HCG diet and HCG injections. Positive results were echoed by Dr. Oz in his review of the HCG diet in 2011 and more recently. Regarding the controversy concerning the effectiveness of the HCG diet, Dr. Oz noted, "..Sometimes the experience of real people does not agree with science."

Dr. Lipman Modernizes the Simeons' Plan with the 800 Calorie HCG Diet

Much of the criticism of the HCG diet has been on the strict food limitations of Dr. Simeons' original 500 calorie diet. Not only is his food plan extremely limited but his other restrictions regarding exercise, supplements, cosmetics and even the administration of the HCG hormone are clearly outdated. Over the past 8 years more "HCG protocols" have been invented to overcome many of these problems. While some have emphasized HCG injection over HCG sublingual drops, most differ by a number of calories and degree of carb restriction.

I will show you how interesting, diverse and modern the HCG Diet can be using numerous newly available foods. You will see how the New 800 Calorie HCG Diet can help you lose weight quickly, safely and still satisfy your hunger and carvings.

This book brings Dr. Simeons' HCG plan into the 21st century. Each one of Dr. Simeons' "directives" has been examined and revised. Simeons' protocol can be done just as effectively without all of the tedium and deprivation of the original 500 calories a day plan.

Phases of the HCG Diet

Dr. Simeons described three phases to his HCG protocol. Phase 1 is the "loading" or binge phase where the dieter consumes a high caloric, high fat intake for 2-3 days while taking HCG.

Phase 2 is the weight loss phase where Dr. Simeons instructed dieters to reduce their intake to 500 calories a day mostly limited to protein and vegetables. Dr. Simeons described Phase 3 as a Stabilization Phase because the purpose is to stabilize your new weight. Most dieters I see elect to skip Phase 1 and begin the diet at the weight loss phase.

800 Calories a Day - NOT 500 Calories a Day

Dr. Simeons wrote: "The diet used in conjunction with HCG must not exceed 500 calories per day, and the way these calories are made up is of utmost importance..." This includes only 200 grams of protein divided between lunch and dinner. For instance, having a breadstick and an apple for breakfast, tea or coffee with only one tablespoon of milk...."

Hundreds of weight loss studies with what is called Very Low-Calorie Diets (VLCD's) have been completed over the past 20 years. They reveal no difference in weight loss between eating 500 or 800 calories a day. In fact, more weight loss and protein sparing have been found at the 800 calorie level. In addition, adding 200-300 calories per day, especially in the form of lean protein for breakfast and a little more protein at the evening meal makes a lot of sense. Here, is an outline of the HCG food plan for 2018 using current products and cooking techniques:

Lean Protein and Fruit for Breakfast-NO SKIPPING BREAKFAST

Dr. Simeons wrote breakfast should consist of "tea or coffee in any quantity without sugar, only one tablespoon of milk...a breadstick or apple ..."

This might appeal to many overweight people who make a habit of skipping breakfast completely. Many researchers believe skipping breakfast may be one of the fundamental reasons for the increase in obesity since Dr. Simeons' time. What is the relation of breakfast to weight loss? Well, breakfast is a simple term which says all about itself in one word. You are breaking the "fast", which you did by not eating for the past 8-12 hours. When you eat breakfast, you are reversing the fasting state while providing energy for the metabolism to function normally. You are also giving yourself a little help in preventing severe hunger at lunch and are helping to give the body a good head start.

Breakfast including proteins such as eggs, high-protein bars or even zero sugar yogurts stabilizes the blood sugar for the rest of day and ensures better choices at lunch. When you skip breakfast, your blood sugar falls throughout the morning and you arrive at lunch not only hungry but with a low blood sugar. Dr. Simeons suggests the use of eggs in his protocol but was concerned because of the high fat (5g/

yolk) found in the yolk. No-fat eggbeaters, another product developed after Dr. Simeons' death, make a great addition to the breakfast choices. It provides high protein, as well as low calories. Portions are easy to control; few people will make more than ½ of a cup of egg beaters. If they do, the calories are so low, it really does not matter. An omelet made from egg beaters and vegetables makes a great nutritious breakfast.

Making bad choices like eating at fast food restaurants or having large lunches that resemble evening meals will come easily if you skip breakfast. Individuals working in schools or offices who skip breakfast and are hungry by lunch are often vulnerable to the "bad choices" that co-workers make and are likely to "go along with the crowd." If you are truly on-the-go, grab an apple, a small piece of cheese, or a protein bar or shake. Something is better than nothing, and you are still following the plan.

More Lean Protein for Lunch and Dinner

"100 grams of lean protein, weighed raw, boiled or grilled with a handful of vegetables and an orange or a few strawberries...dinner is the same four choices as lunch," writes Dr. Simeons in **Pounds and Inches**.

Unfortunately, since Dr. Simeons' time, much has changed in family life. Most women are working, and in some families, the father has two jobs. There is little time to weigh and prepare "100 grams" of protein. In fact, almost no one in the United States refers to food portions by the gram. Instead, food is given in ounces and cups. In addition, although most individuals might be happy with this tiny lunch, they expect more for dinner. Trying to make the meals **equal often does not work**. In this plan larger portions are found in the evening meal, accompanied by unlimited salads and vegetables (with a few exceptions). The addition of vegetables such as cauliflower and zucchini prepared to imitate rice, potatoes, and pasta without the carbs adds variety to the plan.

I also suggest the use of high protein, near zero sugar shakes and bars to be used as meal replacements or even snacks. Most shakes have 15 to 25 grams of protein. Healthy, high protein, low sugar shakes, and bars were unknown to Dr. Simeons.

Three Fruits per Day and Unlimited Vegetables

Dr. Simeons' protocol allows for "an apple, an orange, and a handful of strawberries or ½ grapefruit." The recent low carb craze and the development of the glycemic index have revealed that many more fruits and vegetables can be appropriate, including blueberries, plums, blackberries, raspberries, pears, cherries, peaches and unlimited quantities of salads and many vegetables (There are a few exceptions.) These fruits have low glycemic indices and do not raise the blood sugar or turn to fat. I tell my patients how fast the sugar is absorbed rather than the total amount of sugar that really counts.

Unlimited Zero Calorie, Zero Fat Drinks

In **Pounds and Inches**, Dr. Simeons wrote, "tea, coffee, plain water or mineral water are the only drinks allowed." He adds, "Saccharin or other sweeteners may be used. In many countries, specially prepared unsweetened and low-calorie foods are freely available and some of these can be tentatively used."

Does this mean that artificially sweetened drinks and foods are disallowed or does it reflect the fact that few artificial sweeteners were available in the 1950-60's when Dr. Simeons did his research? The intense debate about the usefulness of artificial sweeteners is reviewed in later chapters. Suffice it to say, for most overweight people and especially diabetics this author has found them useful, safe and effective. Since Dr. Simeons approved of Saccharine and Stevia, might he have approved of Aspartame (NutraSweet, Equal) and Sucralose (Splenda) and Truvia? All of these sugar substitutes are acceptable.

Eliminate the "Binging" and Overeating in the First Few Days

Dr. Simeons wrote in **Pounds and Inches**, "Patients must eat to capacity for about one week before starting treatment; regardless of how much they weigh... they may gain in the process... Normal fat reserves need to be well stocked... Gorging for at least two days must be insisted upon categorically... The subsequent loss is from the abnormal fat deposits only." Telling individuals struggling with their weight and compulsive eating to go out and eat as much fatty food as they are able is at first very appealing, but what is the proof that it leads to more weight loss?

Over the past ten years, I have my patients decide whether to "binge" or start the HCG phase 2 protocol (800 calories) on day one. Interviewing patients during their HCG diet, I am unable to tell which binged and which did not by looking at their hunger or weight loss. Numerous VLCD diet plans have been used in the past twenty years. Not one has advocated such "binging" as a technique to increase weight loss or diminish hunger. All the recent research in overweight individuals indicate their fat cells are already "filled" and "well stocked" due to years of overeating. Adding more fat, if that were even possible, seems to be unnecessary to this author.

Six Week Treatment Plans and Lack of Immunity to HCG

Dr. Simeons wrote, "The reason for limiting a course to 40 injections is that by then some patients may begin to show signs of HCG immunity... we cannot define its mechanism." He goes on to say, "Patients who need 2-3 injections may be injected daily including Sundays..."

Are all of these complicated treatment plans and artificial limitations really necessary? Do people taking HCG administered intramuscularly really get immune to the hormone or is HCG no different than insulin, growth hormone and numerous other naturally occurring hormones where no significant immunity is seen even after years of treatment? Was the HCG immunity Dr. Simeons saw due to the relative impurity in his HCG preparations as compared to current day HCG? Here, are better explanations for the slowdown in weight loss Dr. Simeons observed and interpreted as immunity to HCG:

- The normal response to weight loss is to slow metabolism to prevent further weight loss. Slowdowns are seen in every diet.
- Weight loss is proportional to what a person weighs.
- Dr. Simeons' HCG food plan is limiting and boring. People naturally start cheating which may cause slowdowns.

All of these explanations may play a role in the apparent slow down in weight loss of the Simeons' HCG diet in the past. If a person is doing well on the diet, then there are no reasons to stop, especially if he is taking vitamin and mineral replacements.

Vitamins, Mineral Supplementation is Required and Medications Should Not Be Discontinued

Thyroid Hormone Medication: In **Pounds and Inches**, Dr. Simeons states very emphatically, "We never allow thyroid (replacement) to be taken during treatment. A BMR test (an old-fashioned measure of thyroid function) which is low before treatment is usually found normal after a week or two of treatment." Dr. Simeons was inferring that taking HCG will cause a low thyroid to become normal after a week of treatment! The evidence for that was not presented, and this author does not believe it's possible. Patients that are on thyroid replacement therapy should not stop taking their medications, contrary to what Dr. Simeons wrote. Other Medications: Dr. Simeons wrote, "No medications or cosmetics... may be used without special permission."

I hope the beginning dieter will never follow this bad advice about stopping all medications. It's simply baseless, often dangerous and certainly not necessary. Ask your own physician if you are in doubt.

Vitamin and Mineral Supplements

Dr. Simeons in **Pounds and Inches**, wrote, "Every time they lose a pound of fatty tissue... only the actual fat is burned up, all of the vitamins, the proteins in the blood and the minerals contained in this tissue in abundance are fed back into the body... we have never encountered signs of lack of vitamins who are dieting regularly."

It is true that fat cells contain many nutrients; however most of the nutrients the body needs are not stored primarily in fat cells. Among the fat-soluble vitamins A, D, E, and K, only vitamin K is stored in fat cells. Vitamin A and D are stored in the liver. Water-soluble vitamins B and C are hardly stored at all; they circulate and are excreted in the urine. Vitamin B-12 is stored in the liver. The major storage of calcium and magnesium is in bones rather than fat cells. Current day treatments with VLCD diets add vitamins and minerals as routine without question. It's simple, inexpensive and safe to add multivitamins, sub-lingual Vitamin B12, and oral potassium.

Cosmetics Do Not Stop Weight Loss: Dr. Simeons Was Wrong!

In **Pounds and Inches**, Dr. Simeons spends a great deal of time con-demning cosmetics as interfering with weight loss. He wrote, "When no dietary error is elicited we turn to cosmetics. Most women find it hard to believe that fats, oils, creams and ointments applied to the skin are absorbed and interfere with weight reduction. Just... we find that beauty parlor operators, masseurs and butchers never show sat-isfactory weight loss unless they can avoid fat coming into contact with their skin."

Dr. Simeons cites examples of woman transferring cosmetics and a man with a glass eyeball coming into contact with fatty products thru their skin. He ends, "We are practically averse to those modern cos-metics which contain hormones, as any interference with endocrine regulations during treatment must be absolutely avoided."

Endocrine active substances or hormonally active substances are chemicals that may alter the function of the endocrine system. Al-though a variety of chemicals have been found to disrupt the endo-crine system in studies of laboratory animals at very high doses and in some populations of fish and wildlife, the FDA has found no evidence that ingredients used in current day cosmetic and personal care prod-ucts cause endocrine disruption or alter metabolism in humans. Cos-metics in the United States have been regulated for the past twenty years by the FD&C (Federal Food, Drug, and Cosmetic Act and the Fair Packaging and Labeling Act).

HCG Can Be Taken Effectively Orally As Well As by Injection

Dr. Simeons explains that his HCG can be given only by injection. He wrote, "Once HCG is in solution it is far less stable. It can be kept only a few days at room temperature and longer refrigerated... two inch long needles are used and injected deep intragluteally. The injection should if possible not be given in the superficial fat layers."

There are few current proponents of the Simeons Protocol that call for the HCG to prepared every few days and even fewer that require an injection deep into the buttocks. The latter issue is due to the necessity of having a medical professional perform the daily injections. Dr. Simeons treated patients as inpatients or outpatients in his Rome hospital. The only HCG he used was that extracted from pregnant women's urine. In that setting, it might have been convenient to administer HCG as he indicated. Today, few overweight patients want to see a medical professional daily for a deep intramuscular injection. In addition, the HCG is totally different, it's highly purified, synthetically produced HCG. It's not necessary or practical to prepare HCG daily.

Actually, there is no such thing as "oral" HCG. HCG cannot be swallowed because it's quickly degraded by stomach acids. Like insulin, stomach acids break down the HCG molecule to render it ineffective. Oral HCG really means taking it sublingually (under the tongue.) In the area right under everyone's tongue are a complex set of tiny capillaries which permit rapid absorption of drugs when placed there by an oral syringe. HCG taken sublingually is equally effective as taken intramuscularly. The dose and frequency are increased to lessen any amount of HCG that is inadvertently swallowed. The invention of oral HCG is good news for those that want to avoid injections. If you are taking HCG orally, you need to follow the directions of the manufacturer. In general, most prescription HCG preparations are giving you 250-400 IU. It is usually taken twice a day. Many of the HCG preparations are prepared with bacteriostatic water, alcohol and vegetable glycerin to increase the absorption and keep the HCG stable.

Recently sublingual HCG pills have come to the market. Taken once or twice a day, each pill contains 500 units of HCG. Due to limited testing, I cannot comment on the effectiveness of this preparation.

Menstruation

The HCG can be started at any time in a women's cycle and does not have to be stopped during menstruation. Menstrual periods may become irregular or missed entirely. This is due to the dramatic weight loss, not the HCG and can happen on any weight loss program.

HCG Treatment: How Long? Depends On How Many Pounds You

Need to Lose

You can take the HCG diet for up to a total of 6 weeks without stopping. If you are taking HCG for more than 30 days you need to take daily multi-vitamins, Vitamin B-12 and potassium to prevent possible depletion of these important substances. I suggest a vitamin-like Centrum, Potassium and Vitamin B-12 sublingual tablets or liquid. (All available at CVS, Walgreen's, Wal-Mart, Costco, Target etc).

Stopping the HCG:

You need to continue the food plan for 2 days without the HCG. This is an essential part of the treatment because if you start eating normally as long as there is even a trace of HCG in your body you will gain weight quickly.

Phase 3 HCG:

After phase 2, you should go to the 1100 Calorie High Metabolism Plan outlined in Part 2 of this book.

RICHARD L. LIPMAN M.D.

800 Calorie HCG Diet: Calories, Carbs & Protein

Phase 1: The Binge Phase (Optional)

Most dieters skip Phase 1- the binge or "loading" days. I have seen no difference in hunger or weight loss in those that "binge" and those that do not. If you want to binge here is how: Day # 1 or Days #1 and #2: These are "loading" days wherein one gorges on very high calorie, high-fat foods. HCG is taken twice a day during this period. You should be eating an extra 1000-1500 calories per day. Focus on cheeses, avocados, and heavy creams. If you are doing the binge for only a single day, I suggest adding flax seed oil capsules: take 1200 mg. in divided doses over that day.

Dr. Simeons states that the binge "alerts" the metabolism setting up an atmosphere to burn fat. Dr. Simeons states that it also helps to relieve hunger and other discomforts in the first week of the diet. Many people use the weekend as their loading up days and start the 800 calorie a day plan on a Monday. Here, are some examples of food for binge day(s):

Breakfast: Cream cheese bagel with bacon and sausage, or a ham/cheese omelet. Have some fun, go to IHOP and have some pancakes and load them with all sorts of bad things.

Mid-morning snack: Donut with whipped cream and strawberry jam. Lunch: steak, chicken, potato with sour cream, and a roll with butter and a buttered veggie.

Mid-afternoon snack: Ice cream with Oreos.

Dinner: Pasta such as Fettuccini Alfredo, pizza, cheese garlic bread, and salad with full-fat dressing, of course, cheesecake for dessert. Late night snack: Ice cream or frozen cappuccino.

Once you have fat loaded for one or two days, you will start the restricted calorie diet. Initially, it is common to have hunger cravings, but these will subside between days 5-7. Calories should average about 800-900 per day. You should not skip a meal because it only results in hunger later in the day. An egg, piece of no fat cheese, protein shake, or bar can serve as a meal. Again I see no reason for the binge, but the decision is left to the dieter.

Phase 2: The Weight Loss Phase

The 800 Calorie HCG Diet is designed to follow the principles of the Simeons diet with high protein and minimal carbs but has been modified by following modern-day principles and using current products. Protein is suggested at each meal and often for snacks because of all foods, protein-based foods lead to the most satiety and satisfaction.

Macronutrients in the HCG Diet:

Carbs, Sugar, Protein, and Fat: Sugar should be ideally **2 grams per food portion** or less but up to 4 grams is permitted once a day on a single food item. Fat should be **4 grams ideally or less per item**. Fat in this diet plan is much less important than carbs and sugar. The total of ideal sugar and fat is 2 + 4 = 6 grams per item. All of these represent a single serving. **Protein should be as high as possible**. Foods that have protein of 10 grams or more will make you full. Net carbs are the total carbs less the fiber and sugar alcohols; they should be 10 grams or less per item. Higher carbs or sugars will stop the important fat burning seen in the HCG diet as the body switches from using fat for metabolism to using carbs.

Using the nutrition label you are able to make the best food choices. Here are some of the guidelines you can follow.

"2 + 4" Rule for Picking Best HCG Foods

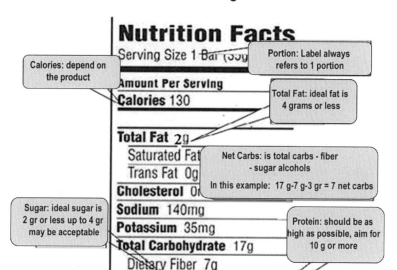

Daily Calories: Women: 800 calories a day, Men: 800-900 calories a day

Men can eat up to 900 calories a day and be successful while women require 100 to 150 calories a day or less. Variety is the key to success. You should expect variation in daily calories. Use the colored food menus in the next chapter to guide you with calories, choices, portions, and preparation. If you follow the food menus, you will end up with the correct calories per day without having to actually count the calories. Of course, you can use free online Apps such as Lose-It or My Fitness Pal to help you.

Calories count especially with portions of protein. Vegetables are unlimited (except no carrots, corn or peas), and there are 3 medium size fruits a day. The packaged food products presented in the menu were carefully selected based on calories, sugar, fat, total carb content and ease of portion control. Substitutions are acceptable if they are comparable. Often they are not. Skipping meals is not a good idea. Substitute a protein shake or bar if you have no time to prepare the foods suggested. Many low calories, zero sugar, low-fat snacks are presented. Ease of portion control is important in meal/snack choices.

Daily Carbs and Sugar: up to 40-50 grams of net carbs/day

The typical US diet of 2000 calories a day consists of 200-300 grams of carbs a day. The American Diabetes Association states that less than 120 carbs a day represent a "low-carb diet." The ultra low- carb Atkins Diet starts off with 20-25 grams of net carbs a day. The Simeons protocol allowed about 30-40 carbs/day. Again as in the daily calories, the food choices and portions on the daily food menus will help you to choose the best carbs without exceeding the daily maximum. Most of the carbs will come from the fruits and vegetables. Rather than using net carbs for fruits, we use the glycemic index always choosing fruits with the lowest index such as berries.

In the 800 Calorie HCG Diet, the allowable net carbs per day should be 40-50 grams or less. The lower the carbs the greater the weight loss. Ultra low carb diets (< 50 grams/day) are associated with less hunger. The table below will help you see the relationship between net carbs intake and weight loss. Note that as daily net carbs are decreased from 300 grams a day, weight loss per week gradually rises. Individuals eating less than 50 grams of net carbs a day can lose more than 4 lbs a week.

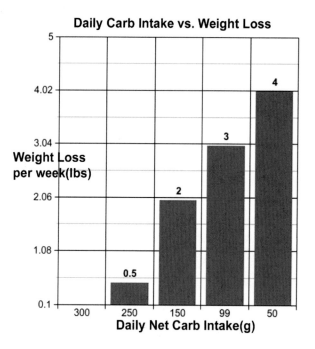

Daily Carb Intake vs. Weight Loss

Vegetables: unlimited quantities with a few exceptions

Most vegetables are very low in net carbs, calories, and protein. In this diet plan, all vegetables are unlimited except for avocados, butternut and acorn squash, peas, corn, and carrots. They are discouraged because of the higher amount of carbs. Many dieters eat almost unlimited portions of avocados thinking they are "healthy." Maybe the fat is "healthy", but overall they are high in calories with difficult portion control. Unlike Dr. Simeons' diet, you can eat the same vegetables for both meals. In the following table avoid vegetables label in red, they have too many calories and/or carbs.

Vegetables : Calories Net Carbs^ Protein

Vegetables and serving size	Calories	Total C	Net C	Protein
Asparagus, cooked, 1/2 cup	20	3.7	2	2
Avocado, 3.5 ounces#	167	8.64	1.8	2
Broccoli, cooked, 1/2 cup	27	5.6	3	1.87
Carrots, baby, 3.5 ounces, raw	35	8.2	5.3	0.6
Cauliflower, 1 cup cooked	34	6.75	1.85	2.9
Celery, 2 ounces, raw	9	1.6	0.67	0.39
Cucumber, 1 ounce, raw	4	1	0.9	0.18
Black Beans, 1 cup cooked*	227	41	26	15
Green beans, cooked, 1/2 cup	22	4.9	2.9	1.18
Mashroom, button, 1 ounce	6	0.91	0.61	0.87
Onion, green 1/2 cup, chopped	16	3.7	2.3	0.92
Corn, 1 med ear (6-7")	77	17	15	3
Pepper, Sweet, green, 1 ounce	6	17	15	0.2
Pickles, dill, 1 ounce	7	1.5	1	0.3
Romanie lettuce, 1 ounce	5	0.9	0.3	0.3
Butterhead lettuce, 1 ounce	4	0.7	0.4	0.4
Shallots, raw, chopped, 1 oz	20	4.7	4	0.7
Snow peas, 1/2 cup, cooked	34	5.6	3.4	2.6
Spinach, 5 oz raw	33	5	2	4
Squash, Acorn, baked, 1 cup	115	30	21	2.3
Squash, Butternut, 1 cup	82	21.5	15	1.8
Squash, Summer, 1 cup	41	6.8	4.8	1.8
Squash, Spaghetti, 1 cup	42	10	8	1
Tomato, raw, 1 ounce	5	1	0.7	0.2

^Total C- Total Carbs, Net C- net carbs

*Black beans: high calories, high carbs, despite high protein, fiber

Avocado: high calories, low protein, low carbs

Fruits: Calories, Carbs, Glycemic Index - 3 choices a day

Fruits are more difficult to understand in the 800 calorie HCG diet than any other food. Many have a lot of carbs and sugar. However, it's not the actual absolute amount of sugar that counts, it's the amount of sugar that is absorbed from the stomach and raises the blood sugar. We use the glycemic index to express this concept. Foods that have a

high glycemic index (GI) above 70% such as sugar, car
the blood sugar quickly and then quickly turn to fat
leased from the pancreas. Foods that have a low glyc
or less, have little influence on the blood sugar and ...
able in the HCG diet. When choosing fruits we look at the calories,
GI, and the ease of portion control. Suggestions are presented in the
table below. *Avoid fruits highlighted in red on the table. They have*
too many calories, carbs or a high glycemic index. Some have portion
control problems like grapes and raisins.

Fruit Choices for 800 Calorie HCG Diet

	size	calories	sugar(g)	total carbs(g)	glycemic index
Apple	Large	80	25	34	36
Banana	Med	110	19	30	53
Blackberries	1 Cup	90	6	13	27
Blueberries	1 Cup	85	11	27	30
Cantaloupe	1 cup	50	11	12	65
Cherries	1 Cup	90	16	26	40
Dates	5-6 dates	200	25	30	72
Grapefruit	1/2 Med	60	11	15	25
Grapes	3/4 Cup	45	20	23	43
Orange	Med	70	14	19	43
Peach	Med	40	13	15	28
Pear	Med	65	16	26	36
Pineapple	2-3 rings	60	16	22	46
Raisins	1/4 Cup	140	29	31	64
Raspberries	1 Cup	60	12	17	27
Waterlemon	2 Cups	118	20	21	72

You can see how most of the carbs will come from the fruits since
the vegetables have net carbs of 1-2 grams. To make choices simpler,
use the Fruit Menu in the next chapter for choices and portions.

Proteins: 100-150 grams per day or 25-30 grams of protein per meal

Proteins, which are made up of chains of amino acids, are essential
nutrients for the human body. In fact, the word "protein" comes from
the Greek word - protos which means "first." You need protein to build

scle, skin, brain and even bones. They are not only the building locks of all tissues in the body but they can be used as a fuel source like fat. Unlike carbs, which are not essential for our body, protein and fat are a vital part of our diet. Without these two nutrients, we would simply not survive.

The Institute of Medicine had established the Recommended Dietary Allowance (RDA) **for** protein as 0.36 grams of protein per pound of body weight. The RDA is the amount of a nutrient you need to meet your basic nutritional requirements. In a sense, it's the minimum amount you need to keep from getting sick and **not** the specific amount you should eat every day. The actual amount depends on your gender and activity levels. A man, who weighs 175 lbs, would need a minimum of 165 lb x 0.36 or 59 grams of protein per day. In general, the RDA of protein for women is a **minimum** 46 grams per day and for men 59 grams per day.

There's a misunderstanding not only among the public but also somewhat among physicians and dieticians: "People think we all eat too much protein." The issue was reviewed by 40 nutritional scientists in Washington DC and published in Journal of Clinical Nutrition. The scientists found that people were eating too **little** protein rather than too much.

They recommended twice the RDA or even higher so that the protein roughly counted for 15-25% of daily calories. The 175 lb man would seek .8 x 175 lb or 140 g of protein per day. In fact, many weight loss studies have shown greater weight loss when daily protein is from 100 to 150 grams per day! Emerging science suggests a protein intake of 25-30 grams per meal. This should be even higher in people exercising. The higher the protein, the less hungry and the faster the weight loss. The problem is not **to exceed** the calorie allotment for the day. It's easy to quickly raise the calories when eating cheese, beef, and pork because the fats and subsequently the calories are high as compared to chicken, fish or eggs.

Safety of high protein: Contrary to popular opinion high protein does not damage the kidneys or liver and only has to be restricted in people with liver or kidney failure.

Source of Protein for Diet*

	Protein (g)	Portion	Calories
Vegetables			
spinach	5 g	1 cup	41
mushrooms	6 g	1/2 cup	30
artichokes	4 g	1 cup	75
broccoil	3 g	1 cup	10
Animal Proteins			
lean beef	26 g	4 oz	133
pork	24 g	4 oz	124
fish	16 g	3 oz	77
chicken/turkey	16g	3 oz	73
egg	6 g	1 egg	65
High Protein Bars/Shakes	20-30 g	1	140-190

Nuts & seeds have too many calories for weight loss
Beans have high protein but too many carbs

The HCG diet is based on protein at each meal and even for snacks (protein bars, protein shakes, and low-fat cheese). Most dieters forget there is protein in vegetables as well. Note in the table the highest proteins are found in the "animal proteins." Only limited protein is found in the vegetable groups. Fruits have little to no protein. Protein levels in nuts and seeds are low (3 g of protein/100 calorie of nuts-about 12 almonds.) Red and black beans may have high protein but too many carbs for the HCG diet.

Veggie Carbs: Cauliflower Rice & Potatoes, Zucchini Pasta--add variety

Many struggling to lose weight eat rice, pasta, and potatoes daily. I call these the "major carbs" as opposed to bread, fruits, cookies, chips which I call "minor carbs." All have few nutrients, high calories, and high carbs. Rice and pasta have more than 200 calories per cup and 40-46 g of carbs. Any of these carbs including potatoes will stop fat burning and the STOP weight loss on the HCG Diet. Quickly broken down into simple sugars in the stomach they raise blood sugar and are converted to fat and produce hunger. All of these major carbs including white and brown rice and pasta, potatoes, quinoa, red and black beans and even sweet potatoes need to be avoided in this plan. Here are some other risks associated with eating these major carb:

- Increased sugar cravings and hunger
- High blood sugar spikes which later result in lethargy and fatigue
- Mental Fog
- Feeling full and uncomfortable after meals
- Stomach issues such as flatulence, belching and bloating
- Mood swings
- Increase sugar can lead to diabetes and cardiovascular disease
- Increased carbs leads to elevated LDL cholesterol
- Elevated sugar increases risks for cancer

Good Alternatives to Rice, Pasta, Potatoes

The recent low carb craze in the weight loss industry has encouraged the development of ultra-low carb and low-calorie substitutes for these carbs. One cup of cauliflower has 25 calories and 1-2 carbs as compared to white rice that has 220 calories and 45 grams of carbs per cup. You can purchase them frozen in your local supermarket. Many supermarkets including Costco sell fresh zucchini and fresh cauliflower already prepared to resemble rice or even mashed potatoes. These new products include:

Frozen Products Available at Local Supermarkets
Cauliflower Rice
Cauliflower Mashed (tastes like potatoes)

Zucchini-Lentil Pasta
Cauliflower: pizza crust, flatbreads, tots
Broccoli Tots
Spaghetti Squash
Veggie tots (made of corn or cauliflower)

Fresh Products

Cauliflower Spirals
Squash Spirals (many types)

Refrigerated Noodle Products

These products are made from the Konjac Yam from Japan and are sold in plastic pouches. They are translucent, gelatinous noodle with a slightly fishy odor. A 4-ounce serving of House Foods Tofu Shirataki Spaghetti contains 10 calories, .5 grams of fat, .3 grams of carbohydrates and less than 1 gram of protein. They come in many forms and are substitutes for pasta and rice and include:

Miracle Noodles
Shirataki noodles
Pasta Zero

Here is what some of these frozen products look like and a home spiralizer:

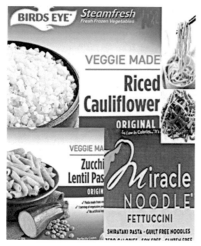
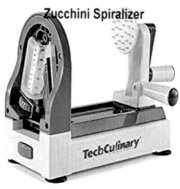
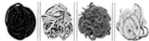

Summary of Food and Drinks for 800 Calorie HCG Diet in Phase 2

Foods and Drinks Allowed:

Download and print full list: https://bestbuyhcg.com/bbhcg_cdl_files/HCG-Shopping-List.pdf

Proteins: eggs & egg beaters, beef (lean) chicken breast (skinless), white meat of turkey, turkey burgers, sea bass, sole, flounder, halibut, grouper, snapper, tilapia, perch, oysters, lobster, crab, shrimp, scallops, clams, **Luncheon meats:** turkey, chicken, ham, roast beef

Pre-packed protein: white albacore tuna, chicken in packs or cans, Tyson or Perdue Cooked Chicken Strips

Protein Bars & Shakes: (Calories 170 or less, 1-2 g sugar, 10 g protein or more): Quest, Extend, Atkins, Detour, Pure Protein, EAS, Muscle Milk (non- dairy),

Vegetables: unlimited - spinach, lettuce, cucumbers, cabbage, tomatoes, asparagus, onions, celery, broccoli, radishes, kale, pumpkin, Brussels sprouts, green beans, mushrooms, peppers, zucchini, cauliflower, dill pickles, bean sprouts, beets, eggplant, bok choy, New Frozen Rice Cauliflower, Cauliflower potatoes, Zucchini Pasta.

Teas and beverages: diet sodas, green tea, black tea, carbonated water, coffee, tea, crystal light, Diet V-8 Splash, Powerade Zero (like Gatorade with no sugar), coffemate (original), Milk: the lowest cow's milk is Fairlife No Fat: (1 cup= 80 calories, 6g sugar, 13g protein). An alternative is unsweetened Almond Milk at 35 calories a cup and no sugar. Small quantities of no fat cow's milk or soy milk are acceptable.

Salad dressings: Wishbone or Ken's low-fat dressings, Walden Farms No Calorie-No Fat-No sugar dressing, olive oil sprays NO OLIVE OIL (too many calories)

Condiments and additives: one tablespoon of fat free half and half, Equal, Splenda, Stevia, Truvia, Heinz reduced sugar Ketchup, soy sauce, Tabasco, Picante, horseradish, PAM and other no-calorie aerosol based cooking sprays, pickles, olives, sugar free salsa, Coconut Oil

Spray, I Can't Believe It's Not Butter or Smart Balance m
garine spray, NO BUTTER

Seasonings: unlimited - lemon, garlic, thyme, parsley, plum vii.
apple cider vinegar, sea salt, basil, pepper, balsamic vinegar, garlic sait

Noodles: Miracle noodles, Zucchini Pasta, Shirataki noodles (usually found in the produce section of supermarket since package needs
to be refrigerated).

Crackers: (3 a day) Melba toasts, Grissini breadsticks, Wasa, Finn,
Gilda toasts, Flatout Light wrap, Tortilla Factory (a no sugar, no fat,
high protein wrap)

Snacks: (see food plan for choices, all very low sugar, and low fat)
Zero sugar Jell-O & chocolate pudding, no-fat cheese, Soy or Quest
Protein Chips, Walden Farms Spreads, International Coffees, Murray
Sugar- free cookies, Sugar-free popsicles, Philly Swirls, no sugar low-
fat yogurt from Dannon, No-fat Polly-O string cheese, No-fat Baby Bell
Cheese

Hard to Find Products:

The shopping list gives the best brands. However, some might be
not available in all parts of the country. Here is what to look for to find
a comparable brand:

- Low sugar yogurt: Dannon Carb Control - 45 calories, 2 g sugars, 1.5
  g fats.
- Low sugar, low-fat, high protein shakes and bars: Premier, Atkins,
  Quest, Pure Protein, ONE, Extend, Muscle Milk, EAS- 140 calories
  or more, 0 to 3 sugars, and 25 to 35 g protein.
- Low carb wrap: Mission Low Carb, La Tortilla Factory, and Flatout
  Light- 90 calories, 0 sugar.
- Near Zero calorie salad dressing: Kens No-Fat, Walden Farms: no
  calories, 0 sugar, 0 fat

**Very Limited Foods Due to High Calories and/or Portion Control
Problems:**

In order to keep the calories to 800 calories a day, most dieters on this program limit high-calorie olive oil, butter, peanut butter and even nuts and seeds. Three tablespoons of olive oil for cooking or mayo on a wrap can almost account for half of the day's calories. Grab a handful of nuts and you can add another 200 calories and have little food left to satisfy your hunger. Also very limited is salmon, and mixed meats such as salami.

"No" Foods due to the High Carbs or Sugar

- Carbs: No bread, starches, sugar, rice, pasta, potatoes, Quinoa, black or red beans
- Fruits: No banana, pineapple, grapes, watermelon, mangoes
- Vegetables: No carrots, corn, peas
- Drinks: No juices, regular sodas, glasses of milk (even low fat), small amounts are permitted in coffee, sugar-free almond milk is permitted

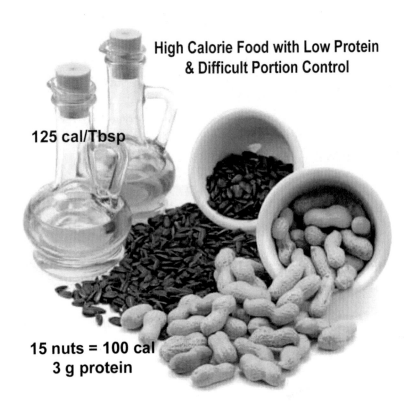

High Calorie Food with Low Protein & Difficult Portion Control

125 cal/Tbsp

**15 nuts = 100 cal
3 g protein**

800 Calorie HCG Diet Daily Meal Menus (Phase 2)

This chapter presents the food menus for the weight loss phase. It includes menus for all meals using thumbnail images to illustrate choices, portions, preparations and calories. You can download a PDF file of the food menus from: https://bestbuyhcg.com/downloads/

Breakfast on the HCG Diet: Calories 160 or less(Phase 2)

For breakfast, you want no more than 160 calories. There are six major choices including choices for sit-down and on-the-go-eating. Breakfast is important in this diet because the proteins not only increase metabolism, they decrease hunger and ensure that you make the best possible food choices at midday. Even if you have little time, you can grab a protein shake, bar or even a portion of cheese.

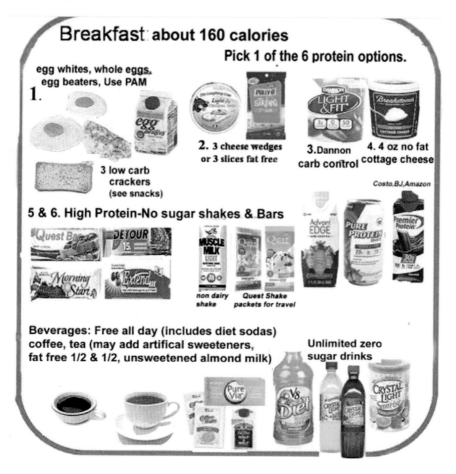

Breakfast: about 160 calories
Pick 1 of the 6 protein options.

1. egg whites, whole eggs, egg beaters, Use PAM
3 low carb crackers (see snacks)

2. 3 cheese wedges or 3 slices fat free

3. Dannon carb control

4. 4 oz no fat cottage cheese
Costco,BJ,Amazon

5 & 6. High Protein-No sugar shakes & Bars
non dairy shake   Quest Shake packets for travel

Beverages: Free all day (includes diet sodas) coffee, tea (may add artifical sweeteners, fat free 1/2 & 1/2, unsweetened almond milk)

Unlimited zero sugar drinks

The above image shows you all of the choices for breakfast. Protein is important for breakfast in order to stabilize the blood sugar. Eggs either 2 whole eggs or (1 yellow and 2 whites), Omelets with vegetables (no cheese or meat) are even better. Add 3 crackers with low-fat cheese. Other selections include low fat-low sugar yogurt, protein bars or protein shakes. Pick one from this group not counting the crackers.

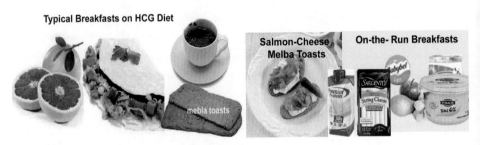

Lunch and Dinner on the HCG Diet

On the 800 calorie HCG diet, there is a large range of food choices for lunch and dinner. Most people I see prefer a smaller lunch and a large dinner. Often lunch is rushed and on-the-run while the evening meal is with family and friends. As long as the calories are equal there is no difference regarding weight loss in having the large meal in the evening vs. at noon. The worst meal timing is to have a large lunch, planning a smaller dinner and then changing your mind and ending up with two large meals! Here are some food menus starting with a small, quick lunch and a larger dinner. Of course, the order of the meals can be reversed.

Food Choices for Smaller Lunch: Calories 250 or less

In the menu below for lunch, the best choices are large salads with protein (2-3 oz.) such as grilled (not fried) chicken or fish with unlimited vegetables or a low-carb wrap filled with vegetables and protein. Remember no mayo or olive oil Avoid nuts and seeds on salads. A high protein (>15-20 g) -low sugar (1-2 sugars or less) bar or shake can replace the foods. Note in the image below in addition to wraps, salads,soups there are yogurts, protein bars and shakes as well as low fat cottage cheese:

Best Choices for Lunch on HCG Diet

Low carb -high fiber wrap
Cut wrap:2/3 for lunch, 1/3 for snack

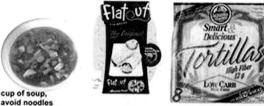

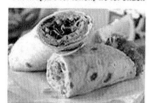

cup of soup,
avoid noodles

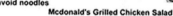

Mcdonald's Grilled Chicken Salad

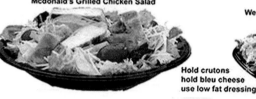

Wendy's Cobb Salad

fill wrap with

tomatoes
veggies
pickles,olives
turkey,tuna
eggs, ham
chicken etc

Hold crutons
hold bleu cheese
use low fat dressing

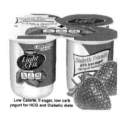

Low Calorie, 0 sugar, low carb
yogurt for HCG and Diabetic diets

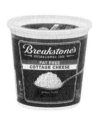

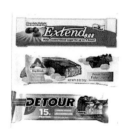

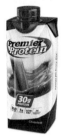

Food Choices for Dinner or Larger Lunch: 300-400 calories or less

There are many choices and combinations in the larger lunch and dinner meal. A high protein bar or shake can be used when the alternati ve is skipping the meal. Non-creamy soups can be used as long as the carbs of the soup such as noodles or rice are not eaten. Otherwise, use a clear soup. Salads and vegetables are unlimited except for beans, carrots, peas, and carrots. Here are some of the guidelines followed by food choices and portions:

• Fish, shrimp, lobster, chicken, beef, and pork- all lean
• Vegetable carbs (such as cauliflower rice)
• Unlimited vegetables (some exceptions)
• Preparation: Grilled, barbequed, sautéed, broiled, baked, steamed
• Condiments: Avoid all cooking oils including olive oil, coconut oil,
   use oil products delivered by spray, avoid butter, Sauces: avoid all
   with sugar

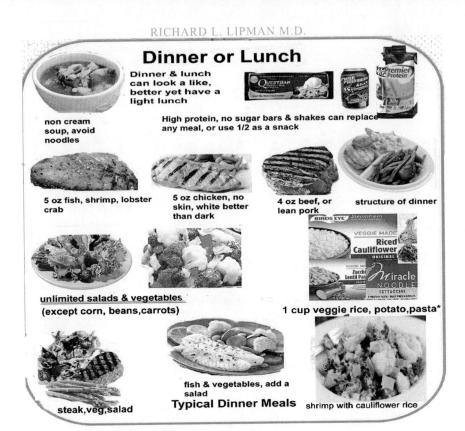

Fruits on the HCG Diet: 3 a day

Here are the choices for fruits on the 800 calorie HCG diet.

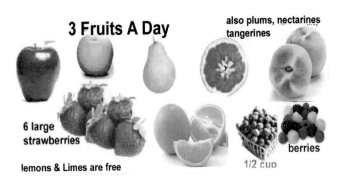

Drinks and Condiments on the HCG Diet

Zero Calorie Drinks

There are unlimited zero calorie drinks on the HCG plan. These include diet sodas, no sugar ice tea, sports drinks such as Powerade Zero, Sparkling waters, Sparkling ICE, Diet Snapple, Propel Zero, Aquafina Flavor Splash, no calorie vitamin waters, and Crystal Light.

Salad Dressings, Condiments

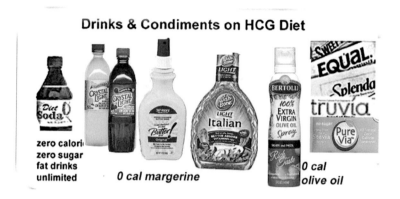

Drinks & Condiments on HCG Diet

zero calorie
zero sugar
fat drinks
unlimited   0 cal margerine   0 cal
                                                          olive oil

Salad dressings have to be very low calorie which ensures they are near zero fat. Vinegar and olive oil, No- Fat Kens Italian Dressing (15 calories/1.5 oz), Wishbone Light Italian, Kraft Fat-Free Catalina, Newman's Own Low Fat, and Walden Farms salad dressings. I Can't Believe It's Not Butter and Smart Balance (both in spray containers and zero calories) are the best margarine selections. There is no difference in artificial sweeteners.

Snacks on the HCG Diet

Why Are Snacks Important in a Weight Loss Program?

Snacks can be an important part of any diet. They can provide energy in the middle of the day or when you exercise. Snacks high in protein and low in sugar prevent low blood sugar reactions and hunger late afternoon that often lead to overeating and binging at the evening meal. High protein snacks besides preventing hunger boost your metabolism.

I have found numerous products over the past 10 years that are appropriate for the HCG diet. My choices were based on:

- **Ease of portion control:** watch bags of chips or large tubs of no sugar ice cream.
- **High protein:** when all else is equal, we chose snacks with high protein. For example, the Halo Ice cream and the Quest Chips both have protein more than 10 grams.
- **Appealing to dieters:** we regularly searched for products that are appealing to patients, usually sweet and salty products. These products satisfy cravings.

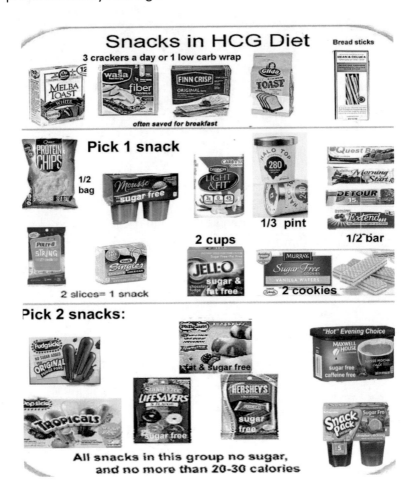

Weight Loss Slow Downs in Phase 2 of HCG Diet

Normal Slowdowns and Plateaus

1. **Last 10 Day Slowdown:** It's normal for weight loss to take a 2 or 3 day pause toward the last 10 days of the plan. Don't let that stop your plan.

2. **4-6 Day Plateau:** Again in the 2nd half of the program you can develop a 4-6 day plateau. Dr. Simeons describes this plateau well: "A plateau always corrects itself, but many patients who have become accustomed to a regular daily loss get unnecessarily worried and begin to fret. No amount of explanation convinces them that a plateau does not mean that they are no longer responding normally to treatment. There are two different approaches to reverse it:

A. Some people try the "Apple Day." An apple-day begins at lunch and continues until just before lunch of the following day: you buy 6 large apples and eat apples whenever you are hungry for the next 24 hours. Six apples are the maximum allowed. No other food is allowed.

B. An alternative is to take a diuretic to get the process moving. This is the easy way, but it needs to be a prescription diuretic. Only do the apple or diuretic after 4 days of stationary weight.

Dietary Errors are the Inevitable Causes of Slow Downs

Most problems are due to mistakes in the diet. A cup of rice or pasta, a glass of tomato juice or some chips can bring the weight loss to a stall. Why does extra food weighing one-ounce increase weight by six ounces?

1. Blood Volume Saturated with Food

Dr. Simeons explained this in the following way (some changes have been made to make the explanation simpler): "Under the influence of HCG the blood is saturated with food and the blood volume has adapted itself so that it can only just accommodate the 500 calories which come from eating. Any extra food however small cannot be accommodated and the blood is therefore forced to increase its volume sufficiently to hold the extra food, which it can only do in a much- diluted form... Thus it is not the weight of what is eaten that plays the determining role but rather the amount of water which the body must retain to accommodate this food... This can be illustrated by mentioning the case of salt. In order to hold one teaspoonful of salt, the body requires one quart of water, as it cannot accommodate salt in any higher concentration. Thus, if a person eats one teaspoonful of salt his weight will go up by more than two pounds, (the weight of 1 quart of water), as soon as this salt is absorbed from his intestine."

2. Eating Sugar and Fat Stops Fat Burning

Any extra sugar or carbs results in stopping the mobilization of the fat and inevitably results in hunger. On the HCG diet, the body is forced to burn stored fat because there is a little intake of sugar) or fat. The body is essentially living on its stored fat.

3. Cosmetics DO NOT Cause Slowdowns!

Every Internet site selling HCG quotes Dr. Simeons' observation: "When no dietary error is elicited we turn to cosmetics. Most women find it hard to believe that fats, oils, creams and ointments applied to the skin are absorbed and interfere with weight reduction just as if they had been eaten. This almost incredible sensitivity to even such very minor increases in nutritional intake is a peculiar feature of the HCG method." ---Personally, I am very skeptical that this problem exists at all with current day cosmetics. I cannot find a single medical study that shows any significant effects of current day cosmetics on human metabolism.

4. Inches Always Comes Before Pounds: The Ratio of Pounds to Inches

Regardless of how many pounds someone has to lose, there is a very constant reduction in the waist which is about 1 - inch decrease in the waistline for every 5 lb. lost. That means if you lose 15 lbs. expect a reduction in your waist of about 3 inches. This does not happen so easily in an ordinary weight loss plan.

Drinking Alcohol on the HCG Diet

Contrary to what many Internet sites selling HCG write, it's possible to drink alcoholic drinks and still lose weight. A healthy lifestyle should be able to accommodate some drinking, especially if you make the right choices. Whether it's healthy to have a single drink every day is still in question. The problem often comes up that many people; especially ones struggling with their weight have difficulties stopping at a single drink. When you are drinking more than one or two drinks a day things begin to change, and it's not just the calories.

Alcohol and Calories

Alcohol causes far more significant problems that might appear by looking at the number of calories in a drink. After all, a glass of wine is only 90 calories, a shot of vodka or whiskey is only 95 calories and a light beer can be as low as 65-75 calories. If it's not the calories, then what is it that makes drinking alcohol and losing weight so difficult?

Alcohol Has "Empty Calories"

There are no nutritional benefits to alcohol. That's not disturbing since we don't expect many health benefits in the first place. We all drink for different reasons. I have never heard some say they drink a beer or a vodka and tonic to improve their health. Many people drink red wine because some people, mostly the French, say it's "healthy" and they think it will prolong their lives and prevent heart disease or strokes. Let's face it, that's just an excuse spouses tell each other when they want to drink. Maybe the Mediterranean lifestyle is healthier, but drinking red wine is only one of the many features of the Mediterranean lifestyle. Most Americans I talk to love to pick the parts of the Mediterranean diet they like such as the wine and discard the rest - like the walking, the small portions and the absence of fatty and salty snacks. It's like picking the parts of the Atkins diet - almost unlimited meat, cheese, and other high-calorie fatty foods, and then sneaking in the bread or pasta. It just doesn't work.

Alcohol & Weight Loss

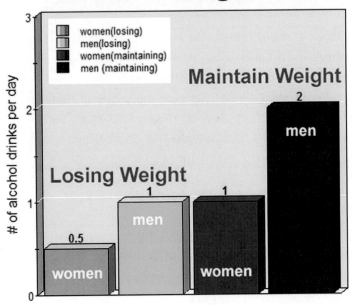

Alcohol Consumption: Men vs. Women

Drinking Alcohol is Often Accompanied by Eating Bad Snacks

In this country, alcohol is accompanied by some high calorie, salty and fatty snacks with absolutely no portion control. It's the chips, crackers, trail mixes, pretzels, nuts, cheese, and wings that add all the calories. Many of the snacks are salty which makes people thirstier, guess what they do? They just drink some more... and it's not water!

Drinking Alcohol Makes Portion Control Difficult and it Stimulates Appetite

Alcohol suppresses control, the brain's ability to say it has had enough - of both alcohol and food. At the same time, it makes people hungrier. The combination of more hunger with less control is very dangerous for some dieters when it comes to picking the right food and watching portion size. Compare the calories after 2 or 3 glasses of wine in a small French restaurant and then try the same in the Cheesecake Factory! Recent studies reveal that drinking a single glass of alcohol is accompanied by an average increase of 120 calories of extra food!

Alcohol and Mixes Have Enormous Calories–Not Acceptable in the HCG Diet

The mixes used in alcoholic drinks are full of sugar. This is a "No-No" in the HCG Diet. Just the mix alone may be twice the calories of the hard liquor. Look at a Pina Colada for 300-400 calories, a Margarita for 300 calories or a simple gin and tonic or vodka and cranberry juice at 250 calories. The alcohol part of all of these drinks was no more than 95 calories. Sugar content easily exceeds 30 grams in some of these mixes.

Alcohol Stops Fat Burning

Alcohol decreases your metabolism and may interfere with HCG's effect on metabolism. When we eat protein, fat, or carbs, some of the food is burned immediately and some of it is stored for future use. However, this does not occur when drinking alcohol. Alcohol is used for metabolism first and is used for energy until all of the alcohol is gone from the bloodstream. It takes the liver 1 hour to clear 1 oz of alcohol. As this is happening, the body cannot use protein, fat or carbs for metabolism and turns them into fat. Less than 5 percent of the alcohol calories you drink are turned into fat. The beer belly occurs not because alcohol is turned into fat but because for long periods of time the alcohol, instead of the recently consumed food or stored fat, is being used for energy.

Alcohol Causes Poor Sleep

Small amounts of alcohol make you feel sleepy but too much alcohol results in poor sleeping, often the result of falls in blood sugar in the middle of the night. Some people wake up and eat. Poor sleeping in itself contributes to weight gain. As we all age, our metabolism slowly decreases. Most of us don't need to further decrease our metabolism by daily alcohol!

How Often Can I Drink Alcoholic Beverages?

It's usually not the calories of alcohol that are the problem in a diet plan, but the other effects that make weight loss difficult. A good plan is to limit drinking to no more than 3 days per week, usually the weekends and special events at the most. Drinking every night, especially for relief of stress, often alone, out of boredom or simply as a habit should be avoided. Most individuals, especially those with slow metabolism due to age, menopause or a sedentary occupation, simply cannot afford to further lower their metabolism every day of the week by the nightly consumption of alcoholic beverages.

Choosing the "Right" Alcoholic Beverage

Deciding to drink alcohol is a very personal choice. Making the best choices in alcohol selection is clearly the most important issue. Similar to the process of choosing foods, the smart dieter keeps the calories as low as possible and avoids high-calorie mixes, often containing lots of carbs that cause hunger, such as juices or tonic. At the same time, he seeks drinks where there is possible "dilution" with zero-calorie fillers. Examples of the latter are soda water mixed with scotch, vodka, or whiskey; and diet cola with rum. Drinking alcohol drinks with zero-calorie "fillers" results in larger volumes of beverages, each having fewer calories. In social situations, it gives the dieter something to hold in his or her hand and feel part of the crowd.

Alcohol and the HCG Diet: Avoid It If You Can... Careful if You Must

After talking with hundreds and hundreds of people on the HCG diet the best advice I can give is this:

- Avoid alcohol - if you can
- 2 or 3 drinks of straight alcohol (vodka, scotch, rum, whiskey, gin etc) per week are probably acceptable.
- Mixes containing sugar and beer (light or not) are not acceptable on the HCG diet.
- White and red wine are acceptable; again 2-3 glasses a week total.
- As in any other weight loss plan: No bad snacks, no drinking for stress, and drink for fun on the weekends. Here are calories in alcohol drinks:

Alcohol Drinks: Calories & Sugar

Drink	Serving	Cal	Sugar(g)
Red wine	5 oz.	100	1
White wine	5 oz.	100	1.5
Champagne	5 oz.	130	2
Light beer	12 oz.	105	2
Regular beer	12 oz.	140	5
Dark beer	12 oz.	170	6-8
Cosmopolitan	3 oz.	165	30
Martini	3 oz.	205	0
Long Island iced tea	8 oz.	400	30
Gin & Tonic	8 oz.	175	22
Rum & Soda	8 oz.	180	28
Margarita	8 oz.	200	5-12
Whiskey Sour	4 oz.	200	5
Gin, Vodka, Tequilla	1.5 oz	95	0
Whiskey, Rum	1.5 oz	95	0

*All straight alcohol drinks have < 1g sugar
Sugar of mixed drinks depend on how prepared

Diabetics Can Do Well on the 800 Calorie HCG Diet

As an endocrinologist and internist, I have been treating overweight diabetics for more than 40 years. Fifteen years ago I began using the 500 calories a day Simeons' HCG diet with injectable HCG. A few diabetic patients were successful, but most did not like taking two injections a day (insulin and HCG) and even more felt that 500 calories a day was simply not enough food for an active lifestyle. The lack of snacks, often important in diabetics, also limited its acceptance. You cannot expect a man who weighs 285 lb and is 6' 3" to have the same energy and food requirements as a woman who weighs 155 lbs and is 5' 2". Some diabetics felt that the amount of protein was too low, especially the total absence of protein at breakfast.

It was also the choice of protein and for some the lack of fruits in the Simeons protocol that was unsatisfactory for most diabetics seeking weight loss. Most diabetics are accustomed to selecting their protein by the calories, carbs, and amount of fat and not by the weight. Dr. Simeons' protocol called for 100 grams of protein at lunch and dinner - not distinguishing between low fat, low-calorie white fish and the high fat, high-calorie beef or pork. Maybe in 1950's Europe the beef was less fatty and lower calorie resulting in fish, chicken, and beef with almost similar calories. However, today the fat differences between proteins result in beef that can be 3 times the calories of an equal portion of white fish.

New Zero Calorie Sweeteners and New Low Carb Foods

It was the low carb craze of the early 2000's that was responsible for making the HCG diet more desirable for overweight diabetics seeking weight loss and control of their blood sugar. Suddenly net carbs, high fiber, glycemic index and new artificial sweeteners were widely available. Every packaged food had this information clearly available. Every packaged food had this information clearly available. Overweight diabetics found that 800 calories was the ideal for women and 900 calories for men.

An example of this was the changes in the breakfast meal. Adding lean protein in the form of eggs, omelets, high protein bars and shakes resulted in a much better acceptance of this diet in people who were not accustomed to skipping meals. Dannon Light and Fit Carb Control yogurt with 2 grams of sugar, 3 net carbs, and 1 gram of fat and only 45 calories combined with fresh fruits is another example of positive changes.

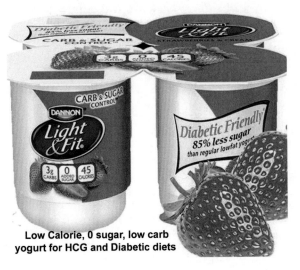

Low Calorie, 0 sugar, low carb yogurt for HCG and Diabetic diets

More recently in 2015, Trader Joes entered the market with fresh and frozen cauliflower rice products. Overwhelming accepted by those adopting a low carb lifestyle these products have quickly spread across the country and now includes cauliflower potatoes and pasta made with Zucchini. Now available in the majority of the grocery store as frozen products these vegetables have been a great addition to the diet of overweight diabetics helping to control both weightand blood sugar.

More Advantages of the 800 Calorie HCG Diet for Diabetics

Food portions are limited in the HCG diet to encourage weight loss - helpful for diabetics especially on medications who have difficulty h weight control.

HCG hormone increases metabolism and fat burning helps diabetics with suppressed metabolism especially when taking diabetic medication. In addition, insulin & other diabetic medication are known to promote fat storage which is reversed by HCG.

HCG Hormone is "natural." It does not interfere with any medication including oral medications, new injectable GLP-1 injections or insulin.

HCG Friendly Foods for overweight diabetics: Here some of the attributes you are looking for in selecting HCG friendly foods that are also desirable for overweight diabetics:

Vegetable Substitues for Rice, Pasa, Potatoes

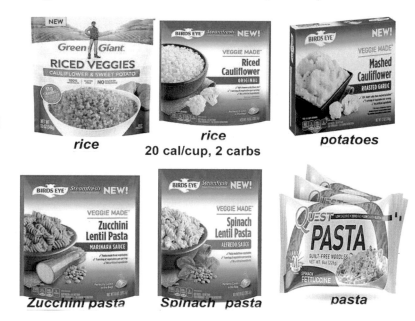

rice

rice
20 cal/cup, 2 carbs

potatoes

Zucchini pasta

Spinach pasta

pasta

Ideal New Products should have these characteristics

- Low in calories
- 2-3 grams of sugar per portion or less
- 3 grams of fat per portion or less
- High protein-low fat when possible.
- Easy portion control.

Vegetarians Are Successful On
The 800 Calorie HCG Diet

Weight loss for vegetarians on the HCG diet can often be a difficult problem. Many vegetarians have difficulty losing weight because of large amounts of carbs and the limited amount of animal proteins they usually consume. With the introduction of many non-animal protein products recently weight loss may not be so difficult. These non-animal proteins can often be substituted for chicken, fish, and meat in the 800 calorie HCG diet. The food pyramid needs to be adjusted for the vegan or vegetarian who uses the HCG diet for weight loss:

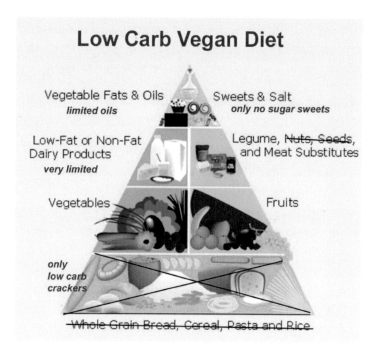

Definitions of Vegetarians and Vegans

The generally accepted definition for vegetarians are individuals who do not eat protein from animals including beef, pork, fish, or chicken but do eat dairy products and eggs. Vegans, like vegetarians, exclude eating animal proteins but take it a step further by excluding all animal by-products including dairy, eggs, honey, rennet, and gelatin (The last 2 products are derived from animals).

Despite all of the low-calorie foods, obesity does exist in the vegetarian population. Few weight loss diets have been tailored for vegans. Although not a vegan diet, Weight Watchers can be adapted to the vegan lifestyle. Since the emphasis is on fruits and vegetables with low points, there is a lot of food. However, it really is not the best choice for weight loss.

Worried About Inadequate Proteins?

If you're worried about not getting enough protein on a vegetarian diet, you may be in for a surprise. Most Americans also do not eat enough protein on any diet. Many people still believe that protein is only available from meat and animal sources and we will all fall over dead without animal protein! Unless you're pregnant or an Olympic bodybuilder, you can eat protein without too much effort.

Weight Loss for Vegetarians on the HCG Diet vs. Common Vegetarian Diet

Weight loss for vegetarians on the 800 calorie HCG diet follows the basics of the HCG diet. This is a high protein, very low-carb diet. It is based on eliminating all sugar and refined carbs such as rice, pasta, potatoes, grains, and sugary snack foods, as well as eliminating as much fat as possible. The problem with the 800 calorie HCG diet for vegetarians is making up for their calorie intake when all carbohydrate products are eliminated. The HCG diet can also be adapted to vegans. However, the true vegan who eats no animal products has some difficulty because of eggs, especially no-fat egg beaters (which are a good source of lean protein in the HCG diet), are not part of the vegan lifestyle.

800 Calorie HCG Diet for Vegetarians

Fruits - 3 per day: apples, peaches, all berries, pears, oranges, grapefruits, tangerines, cantaloupes, nectarines, (limes and lemons are free). Berries portions are ½ cup.

Seasonings: unlimited - lemon, garlic, thyme, parsley, plum vinegar, apple cider vinegar, sea salt, basil, pepper, balsamic vinegar, garlic salt.

Vegetables: unlimited - spinach, lettuce, cucumbers, cabbage, tomatoes, asparagus, onions, celery, broccoli, radishes, kale, Brussels sprouts, green beans, mushrooms, peppers, zucchini, cauliflower, dill pickles, bean sprouts, beets, squash, eggplant, pumpkin.

Teas and beverages: diet sodas, green tea, black tea, carbonated water, coffee, tea, crystal light, Diet V-8 Splash, Lactose-free soy milk or almond milk (permissible in small quantities), Power-Ade Zero (like Gatorade with no sugar).

Salad dressings: Wishbone or Ken's no fat dressing; Walden Farms No-Calorie, No-Fat, No sugar dressing. NO OLIVE OIL.

Condiments and Additives: Equal, Splenda, between Stevia and Truvia, Heinz reduced sugar Ketchup, soy, Tabasco, Picante, horseradish, PAM and other no-calorie aerosol based cooking sprays, pickles, olives, sugar-free salsa, soy mayonnaise

Veggie Carbs & Noodles: Miracle noodles, Shirataki noodles (usually found in produce section of supermarket since they must be kept cold), Zucchini Pasta, Cauliflower rice, and Cauliflower potatoes.

Crackers - 3 per day: Melba toasts, Grissini bread sticks, Wasa, Finn, Gilda toasts, Flat Out Light Wrap (a no sugar, no fat, high protein wrap), La Tortilla Factory Low Carb wraps

Snacks: Soy Crisp Chips, Walden Farms Spreads, Sugar-Free Popsicles, Hummus (watch the amount of olive oil - Weight Watchers has a low calorie, low olive oil recipe), vegetarian cheese.

High Protein Products for Vegans and Vegetarians

This is the food group where the standard HCG diet differs from those who follow the vegan or vegetarian eating principles.

Vegetarian Boca Burger Products: All-American Flame Grilled: 14 g protein

The All-American Flame Grilled Boca Burger contains 120 calories, & 15 g of protein.

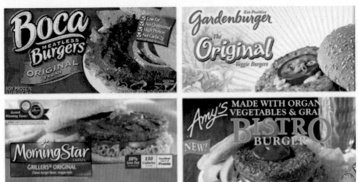

Original Vegan Boca Burger: 13g protein

The Original Vegan Boca Burger contains 70 calories, 5 of which are calories from fat. There is 0.5g of total fat, none of which is saturated fat. It contains no cholesterol, 260mg of sodium, 6g of carbohydrates, 4 of which come from fiber and **13g of protein**. In addition, this burger patty provides 6 percent of the recommended daily value of calcium and 10 percent of the recommended daily value of iron.

Grilled Vegetable Boca Burger: 12 g protein

The Grilled Vegetable Boca Burger contains 80 calories, 10 of which are calories from fat. It contains no cholesterol, 300mg of sodium, 7g of carbohydrates, 4of which come from fiber and 12g of protein. In addition, this burger patty provides 6 percent of the recommended daily value of calcium and 10 percent of the recommended daily value of iron.

Textured Vegetable Protein (TVP®): 13 g protein

TVP is made from 50% soy protein/soy flour or concentrate, but can also be made from cotton seeds, wheat, and oats and no meat products, so it's perfect for those who are on a strict vegetarian diet. TVP® can be purchased flavored with beef, chicken, sausage, and ham. One half cup dry TVP® = 80 calories, 0g fat, 3g sugar, 13g protein, and 7g total carbs.

Tofu and Soy Products: 10 g protein

First used in China around 200 B.C., tofu has long been a staple of Asian cuisine. Tofu soaks up flavors and is best when marinated for at least 30 minutes or served with a flavorful sauce. There are two types of tofu that you'll want to try:

1. **Fresh, Water-Packed Tofu (always refrigerated):** Best for when you want the tofu to hold its shape, such as when baking or grilling

2. **Silken Tofu:** Packed in aseptic boxes and usually not refrigerated.

Try firm or extra-firm tofu for baking, grilling, sautéing, and frying and soft or silken tofu for creamy sauces, desserts, and dressings. To give tofu a meatier texture, try freezing it for 2 to 24 hours and then defrosting it. Press the water out of the tofu prior to preparing it. Wrap the tofu in a towel and set something heavy on top of it for at least 20 minutes and it will be ready for marinades, sauces, freezing, and cooking. You may have tried tofu and soy milk before, but what about soy ice cream, soy yogurt, soy nuts or soy cheese? TVP® and tempeh are also protein-rich soy foods. As an added bonus, many brands of tofu and soymilk are fortified with other nutrients that vegetarians and vegans need, such as calcium, iron and vitamin B12. **Protein content:** A half-cup of tofu contains **10 grams** of protein and soy milk contains **7 grams of protein** per cup.

Tempeh: 18 g protein

This traditional Indonesian food is made from fermented soybeans and other grains. Unlike tofu, which is made from soybean milk, tempeh contains whole soybeans, making it denser. Because of its density, tempeh should be braised in a flavorful liquid for at least one hour prior to cooking. It's actually similar to a very firm veggie burger, and, like tofu and seitan, it's quite high in protein and can be prepared in a myriad of ways, making it perfect for vegetarians and vegans. Protein content: Varies by brand, but as a guideline, one serving of tempeh (100 grams) provides about 18 grams of protein (that's even more protein per gram than tofu!) Tempeh is a great alternative for those who don't like tofu.

Seitan: 18 g protein

Seitan is derived from the protein portion of wheat (gluten). It replaces meat in many recipes and works so well that a number of vegetarians avoid it because the texture is too "meaty." When simmered in a traditional broth of soy sauce or tamari, ginger, garlic, and kombu (seaweed), it is called seitan. Others simply call it gluten. Commercially made mixes include Arrowhead Mills' Seitan Quick Mix or any of the Knox Mountain products, which include Wheat Balls, Chicken Wheat, and Not-So-Sausage as well as White Wave and Lightlife Foods.

Ener-G® Egg Replacer™ (an egg substitute for recipes): no protein

Ener-G® Egg Replacer™ is made from non-animal sources and replaces eggs for those on the vegan diet or those who cannot have eggs. Ener-G® Egg Replacer™ greatly simplifies baking and allows you to enjoy a variety of delicious egg-free baked goods. It is not nutritionally the same as eggs, but it does mimic what eggs do in a baking recipe. It works best in recipes made from scratch. It will not make scrambled eggs. Ener-G® Egg Replacer™ may work well in some premade commercial mixes, but not in all of them.

It is made from Potato Starch, Tapioca Flour, Leavening (Calcium Lactate, Calcium Carbonate, Cream of Tartar, Cellulose Gum, and Modified Cellulose. It is 100% egg-free (contains NO eggs nor animal protein), it is also gluten-free, wheat-free, casein-free, dairy-free, yeast-free, soy-free, tree nut-free, peanut-free, sodium-free, cholesterol-free, and it's low in protein. 1- 1/2 teaspoons of dry Ener-G® Egg Replacer™ plus 2 tablespoons of warm water equals one egg. Mix thoroughly before adding to the recipe. One replaced egg contains 15 calories, 0g fat, 5mg sodium, 4g carbohydrates, 0g sugar, and 0g protein.

The Vegg, Vegan "Egg Yolk" Mix: no carbs, 1 g protein

The Vegg, Vegan Egg Yolk is a 100% plant-based egg yolk replacement that contains only natural ingredients and 0g fat. For 2-3 yolks, simply mix 1 teaspoon of The Vegg with 1/4 cup of water in a blender and blend until smooth. Then, use the mixture as you would traditional eggs. You can use it in any recipe that calls for egg yolks such as soups and dressings. It also makes delicious tofu scrambles. Since it has only 1 gram of protein it cannot substitute for the protein in eggs.

Vegetarian Cheese: Protein varies from 3 to 7 g per slice

Cheese can be made with or without rennet (which is derived from the stomach tissue of a slaughtered calf). This discussion is about those cheeses which are made without the use of rennet. Today, more and more cheeses are made with "microbial enzymes", which are widely used in the industry because they are a consistent and inexpensive coagulant. All labels should be read carefully. Brands include Land-o-Lakes, Cali-fornia Select, Cabot, Boars Head, and many more.

Shopping for Vegan and Vegetarian Products on the HCG Diet

You must always read labels when shopping for vegan and vege-tarian products on the HCG Diet. What appears as the perfect vegan product might have too much sugar, starch, or fat for the HCG diet. Remember, no sugar, grains, pasta, rice or potatoes - even if they ap-pear low carb and "healthy". You can find a wide variety of vegan and vegetarian foods at Amazon.com, which is especially convenient if the supermarkets near you have a limited selection. You can also find veg-etarian products and retailers on The Vegetarian Resource Group at http://www.vrg.org/links/products.htm.

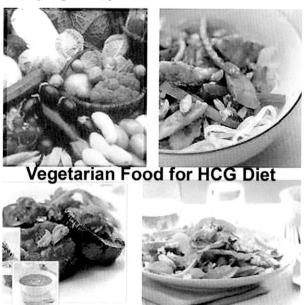

Vegetarian Food for HCG Diet

Exercise on the HCG Plan

Many people are confused when it comes to exercise and the HCG diet. Do you need to exercise? If so, how much should you exercise? What kind of exercise do you need to do? Here is what you need to know about exercise and the HCG diet.

High-intensity workouts on the HCG diet are not recommended because your body has little carbohydrates stored in the form of glycogen in the liver and muscle. Lifting heavy weights, cardiovascular workouts like running or high-intensity step aerobics, or circuit training require large amounts of carbs that you simply do not have available. Attempting these exercise results in rapid dehydration and hypoglycemia (low blood sugar). The result is weakness and a feeling you are going to pass out. This often occurs late in the afternoon.

How Carbohydrates Fuel Exercise

In the HCG diet, you will markedly reduce your carbohydrate calories, your body will start to use up these glycogen stores. Low glycogen forces your body to switch to using more body fat for energy and begin converting amino acids from proteins to fuel. This is the source of the remarkable weight loss in the HCG diet. This often makes intense exercise very difficult. Here's why:

Carbs provide the energy that is needed for exercise. Once eaten, carbohydrates break down into smaller sugars (glucose, fructose, and galactose) that get absorbed and used as energy. Any glucose not needed right away gets stored in the muscles and the liver in the form of glycogen. It's thought that the body can store up to 2000 carbohydrate calories in muscles (15 grams of carbohydrates per 2.2 lbs. body weight). Glycogen is the source of energy most often used for exercise because it is immediately accessible from muscle and liver. The amount of carbohydrate you eat determines the amount of glycogen stored in the liver and muscles, which in turn greatly affects your ability to exercise.

During depletion, from a diet, exercise or a combination, you use up the stored carbohydrates. There is enough stored glycogen for 30-80 minutes of exercise, depending upon the intensity. It takes less than 24 hours of fasting to completely drain your liver glycogen stores. Carbohydrates are the brain and muscle's fuel, so your body needs to use carbs even while you sleep. A glycogen drain will make you may feel listless and uninterested in exercising. That's why in the HCG diet you need to space your exercise out throughout the week. A few days off is needed for your body to recharge the glycogen stores.

What is the Role of Exercise in the HCG Program or any Other Weight Loss Program?

Gary Taubes wrote in Good Calories, Bad Calories (2007): "In the past few years, a series of authoritative reports have advocated ever more physical activity for adults - now up to ninety minutes per day of moderate-intensity exercise - precisely because the evidence in support of the hypothesis is so unimpressive... No substantial evidence, in fact, supports this recommendation for weight loss or maintenance."

In his groundbreaking study published in early 2007, Dr. Ravussin notes physical exercise plays a minor role in weight loss. In a very well controlled study, overweight people who were restricting their calories but did not exercise lost almost the same amount of weight (about 10% of their body weight) compared to those who were restricting their calories AND exercising. Dr. Ravussin adds that exercise can "produce health benefits," such as improvements in blood sugar and aerobic fitness, which do protect against heart disease." Dr. Ravussin writes: "It's all about calories; so long as the energy deficit is the same, body weight will decrease in the same way."

In his extensive clinical study published in the Journal of the American Medical Association (JAMA) in 1999, Dr. Anderson proved what many people suspected: overweight individuals do not have to act like athletes or spend hours in a gym to lose weight and become healthy. Dr. Anderson and other researchers emphasize that sedentary, overweight individuals can be successful in their weight loss plans with a simple and a slight increase in the amount of physical activity in their daily lives. Dr. Anderson writes, "Diet plus lifestyle programs were as effective as diet plus aerobic training programs in improving weight, blood pressure, and serum lipids... This is good news for people who dislike vigorous physical activity or believe they lack the time to exercise."

According to Jamy D. Ard from the University of Alabama in Birmingham, gym exercise - even the strenuous type - is not necessary for weight loss or weight maintenance. In 2007 Dr. Ard writes: "At follow-up, 80% of all participants maintained their body weight and 20% had regained weight. The maintainers consumed 384 fewer kcal a day on average than did the regainers. There was no significant difference in physical activity (minutes/day) reported by maintainers and gainers."

Exercise Does Not Remove Local Fat Accumulation

The exercise industry promotes the idea that working out will also help you to sculpt your body. Using the right equipment or doing the right exercises, according to them, will take fat off the love handles, thighs, underarms, and other very specific parts of your body. Men lose their bellies by doing crunches and women lose their muffin tops.

"It may well be true. For the vast majority of individuals, overweight and obesity result from excess calorie consumption and/or inadequate physical activity. But it also seems that the accumulation of fat in humans and animals is determined to a large extent by factors that have little to do with how much we eat or exercise: that is a biologic component." writes Gary Taubes in Good Calories-Bad Calories.

Our genetic structure makes losing specific localized fat deposits very difficult. Exercising is usually ineffective in permanently altering this distribution. Exhausting yourself by doing hundreds of sit-ups to produce those rock-hard abs that will never be seen if covered with a layer of fat.

What Exercise Is Needed on the HCG Diet?

The evidence presented means that if you are already significantly restricting your food intake as in the HCG Diet, adding exercise may have very little effect in assisting your weight loss. Of course, I'd like everyone to strengthen their heart, circulation, and stimulate muscle and bone growth by completing some exercise. It would also be good for your emotional well being. I do not expect you to do physical exercise at levels that would actually make you lose weight. Unless you are a professional athlete or plan to work out like one over the course of at least 3 to 6 months, that goal is achieved much easier by making smarter food and beverages choices.

Discovering the Lifestyle Exercises

Any extra calorie-burning movement, that you can add to your life as a part of your normal daily routine is what I like to call a lifestyle exercise. The concept is to integrate these extra activities in a way that does not disrupt your normal daily routines. This will allow a few extra calories to be burned off and adds some other health benefits to your life. The old saying, "habits are hard to change" can apply to positive as well as negative behavior. In this case, the "habit" we want to incorporate is almost unconscious daily exercise.

Dr. James Hill at the University of Colorado has written extensively on the use of lifestyle exercises for weight loss and maintenance. He advocates walking an additional 2000 steps per day which translate to burning extra 100 calories per day. Dr. Hill writes in 2006 in the Step Diet: "These results were supportive of our hypothesis that small lifestyle changes can be achieved through a family-based program and can prevent weight gain in adults and excessive weight gain in growing overweight children."

The emphasis on what I call lifestyle exercises are both realistic and simple and can be done by just about anybody, anywhere, at any time.

Examples of Lifestyle Exercises Include:

- Taking the stairs instead of the elevator.
- Parking the car at the far reaches of the parking lot.
- Getting off the bus a stop early and walking the distance to your destination.
- Walking or biking on errands.
- Delivering a message in person in an office, instead of by e-mail.

- Walking your dog an extra block.
- Doing yard work.

Some people have enough self-discipline to implement these life-style exercises naturally. However, the majority of people need a more formal plan and something more structured than taking the stairs every day, but less structured than going to the gym four days a week. For a more formal lifestyle exercise program, try walking. Most of us have the equipment to do this with us every day, even when traveling. Walking cost nothing and can take as little as a few minutes. Even walking for ten minutes several times a day can help stimulate weight loss and more importantly will improve your cardiovascular health.

Benefits from Regular Lifestyle Exercises

Lifestyle exercise can actually assist your weight loss and more specifically, help you through plateaus. I'm not talking about two hours in a gym. Instead, the addition of small amounts of physical activity to your daily routine can improve many aspects of your health. Moreover, such improvements can be experienced by virtually everyone, regardless of age, sex, or physical ability. They will not require great commitments or an enormous amount of willpower. The following is some of the additional benefits of regular lifestyle exercises:

Strengthens your cardiovascular system. The term "cardiovascular system" refers to your heart and your blood vessels. Cholesterol buildup in your arteries can cause strokes and heart attacks. Regular physical activities prevent this from happening. Additional benefits of regular exercise include:

1. Lowers the buildup of bad cholesterol (LDL) in arteries by increasing the concentration of good cholesterol (HDL).
2. Prevents the onset of high blood pressure if you are at an increased risk of developing this condition.
3. Lowers your blood pressure if yours is already high, may prevent or manage diabetes.
4. Keeps bones and muscles strong.
5. Regular physical activities are one of the best methods to prevent osteoporosis and strengthen your muscles. Choose lifestyle exer-

cises that bear your body's weight, such as walking and jogging.
6. Can help to break through plateaus.
7. Manages stress and depression
8. Helps you sleep well
9. Prolongs life span

Frequently Asked Questions

Why Has My Weight Loss Stopped?

Nothing is as discouraging for the first time HCG users as having their remarkable weight loss suddenly stop. Here are simple things to do:

- Drink more water; add a glass of green tea
- Cut out American beef - too much fat
- Are you eating lunch meats or cheese with fat?
- Check condiments for sugar
- Check for additives to chicken or beef
- Any new medications?
- Maybe drop one of the fruits
- Try the Apple Day
- Try a little bit of exercise
- Add 2 tablespoons of apple cider vinegar diluted in water

What is HCG and how does it work?

HCG is a hormone naturally produced in the body. It has many functions and is used medically to treat a variety of conditions. It is the pregnancy hormone. This hormone allows the body to metabolize fat and use it as energy for both mother and fetus. This acts as a "fail-safe" mechanism when energy is needed immediately. For weight loss, we use only a very small amount of HCG to capitalize on this same mechanism. Using HCG in this way does not mimic pregnancy; in fact, it can be safely used by both men and women. HCG is extremely safe. Women may experience very high levels during pregnancy with no adverse effects. Currently, there are no known established clinical side effects.

What sets Dr. Lipman's HCG product apart from the rest?

You will not find this product being sold by other companies; it is a proprietary formula using more expensive quality ingredients that work. My HCG Formula drops may not always be the lowest price, but they will always have the highest quality and diet effects.

What is the difference between prescription and nonprescription HCG?

Prescription HCG can be very effective but must be obtained and monitored only by a licensed medical physician and involves a personal encounter.

Is HCG safe for men?

HCG is as safe in men as it is in women. In fact, men get faster results and tend to lose more weight than women.

Why don't pregnant women lose weight?

HCG works to mobilize fat for utilization by the body only when there is a significant decrease in calories and fat. For weight loss, a very low-calorie diet of all the right foods is used to trigger HCG to help rid the body of fat.

Will metabolism slow down on a very low-calorie diet?

It is true that normally when cutting back on calories and fat, our body stores fat and our metabolism slows down. This happens because fat is really a lifesaving source of stored energy. When a very low-calorie diet is used in conjunction with the HCG, the hormone signals the body to used stored fat for energy. This will eliminate excess fat reserves. It is a natural process, so no ill effects on your metabolism will result. The HCG keeps the body from going into starvation mode and holding onto fat as it resets your metabolism.

Wouldn't I lose the same amount of weight eating a very low-calorie diet without HCG?

You can lose weight simply by eating fewer calories and carbs, but because the body stores fat during times of deprivation, you will most likely lose muscle and bone before fat. This causes cellular metabolism to slow down, so in the long run, it would make gaining weight easier, as well as decreased bone density and muscle mass. By using HCG with the low-calorie diet, extra fat is mobilized for energy and the rest is eliminated. The low-calorie diet is vital in preventing immediate refilling of emptied fat cells. You benefit by preferentially getting rid of excess fat without affecting your bone and muscle.

The HCG diet is very low calorie, will I get hungry?

It is common to feel mild hunger during the first few days. This will pass, and by the second week, you will find your servings to be satisfying. HCG mobilizes fat and makes it available to the body as an energy source, naturally reducing appetite. Adding 20-25 grams of protein at each meal and often as snacks eliminate most of the hunger. In addition, the new vegetable-based carb like foods can add a lot of food without many calories or carbs. The makes the meals more satisfying.

Will HCG interfere with any medications I am currently taking? What about birth control pills or Depo-Provera injections?

No interactions, you are free to take your usual medications.

What about pregnancy and taking HCG?

If you are pregnant or become pregnant during the HCG diet, STOP taking HCG and consult your physician.

How much weight can I expect to lose on the program?

Some people will lose up to 30 pounds, other will lose less. Everyone is different. It depends on many factors including how much excess weight you have, your age and gender and starting weight. Often, people lose 7-14 lbs in the first week. People that have recently dieted will also lose weight slower since the metabolism has already slowed down. The following graph demonstrates how men lose faster than women and younger people lose faster than older people. The graph shows the average weight loss per week during the first 3 weeks of the HCG diet.

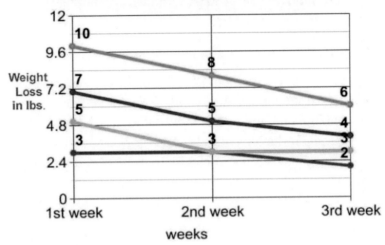

Expected Weekly Weight Loss On HCG

- Green: under 59 males with 40 lbs. to lose
- Purple: over 60 males with 40 lbs. to lose; women under 59 with 40 lbs. to lose
- Orange: under 59 males with 20 lbs. to lose; women over 59 with 40 lbs. to lose
- Brown: Women with 10 punds to loose

Does the weight loss slow down after the first two weeks?

Many times there is a large amount of weight loss in the first week, then a plateau or leveling off of weight loss. This does not mean that your weight loss has stopped. Typically, inches are being lost continuously while on the program, and after a period of time dieters will experience another large drop on the scale. Weight loss is thus achieved in this stair-step fashion.

Is it ok to skip a meal or protein at one of my meals?

NO, you should not skip meals because you will end up with a low blood sugar, become weak and dizzy and perhaps eat more. A protein bar or shake can substitute for a meal.

Do I have to take vitamins while doing this diet?

A good multi-vitamin helps, however, make sure it is sugar-free and has no fat-soluble ingredients like fish oils. Potassium is also good especially if you experience leg cramps, which can be common while on this diet.

Is it normal to get a headache during the first week?

Some people may experience light headaches during the first week. This is the result of your body releasing fat cells very rapidly and the fact you will be going through a major detox. You may take an Aspirin or Tylenol as long as it's not sugar-coated.

Secrets and Tips About the HCG Diet

Ketone Testing in the HCG Diet

Ketones are a normal product of fat metabolism. When fat stores are used for fuel as in the HCG diet, ketones are produced in the liver which passes thru the blood into the lung, kidney, and urine. These ketones come in three common forms; acetoacetate, beta-hydroxy-butyrate, and acetone. In large quantities, they are removed from the body in the urine or through exhalation.

It's the acetone in the breath that causes the unusual fruity smell to the breath of a dieter in ketosis. Ketones are not only expelled by the lung but passed through the kidney and are excreted in the urine. The urine can be tested for ketones using ketone test strips. These strips are small plastic strips that have an absorptive pad on the end that change color when ketones are in the urine. The strip is dipped into the first- morning urine, wait 15 seconds and compare the color change. Any color change indicates fat burning. Don't worry about how dark your strip is. Some low carb dieters NEVER show trace ketones, yet they burn fat and lose weight. Don't get hung up on the strips; they're just a guide. You can buy a full bottle of Keto Strips at any pharmacy, usually in the diabetic supplies.

Ketone Testing in HCG Diet

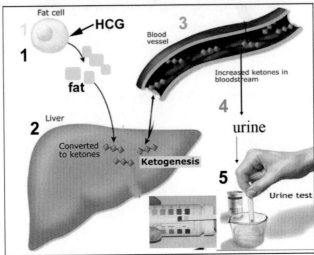

1. Fat cells broken down by HCG
2. Fat is released, goes to liver & forms ketones
3.- 4 Ketones go to blood then to kidney & urine
5. Ketones in urine turn keto strip purple

1. Keto Testing Helps You Avoid Making Food Mistakes:

Keto testing tells you if you are making mistakes and eating too many carbs. It takes 3-4 days in phase 2 to notice a change in the color of the keto strip. This means that your calories, carb, and sugar levels are very low(less than 75 g of carbs/day) and you are burning your stored fat for fuel. Any change in color is a sign of fat burning. If you are losing weight and are not hungry and your strip shows light purple and you wake up the next morning and the strip shows no color change, then you probably ate or drank something the day before with sugar, such as sauce on your meat, sugar in a salad dressing, a dessert, or sugar in your coffee.

2. Ketone Testing Helps You Add New Foods:

One of the criticisms of the HCG diet has been the lack of variety especially in snacks, the boredom, the need to do considerable food preparation and the failure to include many new products. Many new products we have today were not available to Dr. Simeons. The daily food plan contains many foods and products which were discovered by speaking to my patients on the HCG diet, monitoring their hunger and ketosis while they added new products.

HCG Side Effects vs. Side Effects of HCG Food Plan

HCG is a natural substance produced in the human body - there is an only slight possibility of unwanted side effects from the HCG itself. A pregnant woman makes more than 1 million units of HCG a day for 9 months. The HCG dose for injection is 125 units, and the oral dose is slightly higher. Since there is so little HCG (pregnant women make more than 2000 times as much in a single day and are exposed to this dose for 9 months with no side effects), one finds very few side effects taking these small quantities HCG.

HCG signals the hypothalamus (area of the brain that affects metabolism and appetite) to mobilize fat stores. In pregnancy, this helps the body bring nutrients into the placenta, fueling the fetus with the energy to grow. This fat burning is the main effect of HCG in the human body. Side effects of HCG use are uncommon. Most of the side effects are due to the very significant change in foods and include: headaches, irritability, restlessness, slight water retention, constipation, weakness and fatigue and low blood sugar reactions (usually seen when skipping meals or attempting very rigorous exercise.)

Constipation in the HCG Diet is from the Food Change - Not the HCG Hormone

If you have a tendency toward constipation, the HCG food plan will be more likely to make it worse. Constipation may even occur regardless of whether you have had this problem before. There are many reasons for constipation including lack of fat, fruit, and fibers (from grain products) in food and not enough water intake. Remember, any decrease in food intake leads to the longer transit time for food in the small and large bowel and a decrease in motility of the colon. This causes more time for water absorption and results in even further constipation as stools become hard and dry.

Eating a large number of green vegetables may be one of the simplest ways to deal with constipation. At least 3 cups of salad are suggested. However, pale green iceberg lettuce does not have much fiber in it. Try dark green vegetables including steamed vegetables such as broccoli, asparagus, and spinach. These latter vegetables have much more fiber and also lead to more fullness. Increasing your fruits will also help. If you still are constipated add a stool softener like docusate or colace. If constipation continues, then add fiber such as Fibercon (1 - 4 tablets a day, each with a glass of water) or sugar-free Metamucil. Miralax powder is the last resort. Sometimes cutting out the salt in your diet will lead to less fluid retention and stools that are not as dry.

Eight Secrets to Reduce Hunger on the HCG Diet

1. Drink diet soda; carbonation produces fullness.
2. Eat some low-calorie fruits, like strawberries, apples, cherries, peaches.
3. Try a large portion of no-sugar Jell-O, not the tiny little cups, either make it yourself or buy larger portions in the supermarket; you can add fruit to it if you make it yourself.
4. Make some homemade soups: beef or chicken broth, a lot of vegetables, small piece of chicken or fish, and cook.
5. Snack on some extra vegetables, like celery; spray it with the Wishbone Ranch dressing.
6. Buy some no sugar popsicles, scrap two off the stick into a paper bowl, but a dab of Ready Whip - sugar and fat-free whipped cream and enjoy a sundae.
7. Put a low sugar yogurt in a blender with some ice and water, add strawberries or blueberries, add some Splenda.

What Are Most Important Mistakes on HCG Diet?

Mistakes people make on the HCG diet almost always involve food/drinks. The HCG diet is very sensitive. Small variances can mean no or less than desirable weight loss. Often the mistakes are similar to those that people make on any weight loss plan.

1. **Not sticking to the 800 calories** or serving sizes. Protein choices and portions are critical to control the calories in this diet. **American**

beef is significantly fattier than the beef so be careful with the portion. Chicken and fish are always better choices. Foods with higher sugars often creep into the food menus. If in doubt, look at the food label. Sugars should be less than 4 grams per portion.

2. **Not drinking enough water.** You should set as your goal to drink at least a quart of water a day.

3. **Eating beef that is too fatty.** American Beef is very fatty. We suggest using very lean cuts such as London Broil or Round Steak. Even extra lean hamburger can be too fatty, have the butcher cut the fat off a lean steak and have it ground into hamburger meat. Chicken and fish are always better choices.

4. **Cooking with high calorie olive, canola or coconut oil or adding butter and mayo** will add hundreds of unnecessary calories.

5. **Not recognizing hidden sugar in your drinks, seasonings, salad dressings and sauces. Etc.** Sugar is in everything. Avoid foods or drinks with fructose, maltose, lactose, cane juice, galactose, malodextrin, pentose, ribose and sorbitol. Start reading labels, especially on your seasonings. Watch out for words: "no sugar" and "no added sugar" when there is sugar.

6. **Making mistakes in restaurants: The HCG diet can be done when eating out, but watch for the preparation of the food and most important the sauces.**

7. **Taking too many "breaks."** It's acceptable to take a break after a couple of weeks, but not each weekend! "Insidiously, weekend blowouts keep you feeling deprived psychologically", says Sarah Flower, author of The Healthy Lifestyle Diet Cookbook. 'People liken the fun and relaxation of weekends to unhealthy eating,' says Flower. 'They equate their working week with dieting and deprivation, which locks them in the mindset of "good" or "bad" eating. If you feel compelled to overeat every weekend, it suggests the way you're eating most of the time isn't satisfying you,' says Dr. Biffa. 'You're waiting for the weekend when you can enjoy your diet. But the healthy eating should be making you feel better, not be your penance.

8. **Eating "Healthy "** appearing foods in large quantities. Seeds, nuts, olive oil, coconut oil, hummus, pistachios and even avocados con-

tain healthy fat but often have high calories and difficult portion control. Such foods can act as triggers for those with a tendency to overeat. "It's possible to overeat on a healthy diet and as a result not lose weight - or even gain weight ,' says weight loss expert Dr. Biffa." "Being 'healthy' doesn't give people carte blanche to completely ignore calories."

Taking HCG: Oral vs. Injections

In **Pounds and Inches**, Dr. Simeons explained that his HCG must be given only by injection. He wrote, "Once HCG is in solution it is far less stable. It can be kept only a few days at room temperature and longer refrigerated." He added, "Two-inch long needles are used and injected deep into the buttocks. The injection should if possible not be given in the superficial fat layers."

These instructions might have been workable in Dr. Simeons' private clinic in Rome in 1954 but not today There are few current proponents of the Simeons Protocol that require HCG to be prepared every few days and be injected deep into the buttocks. Deep intra-muscular injections are difficult to do yourself and usually are done by a medical professional. Today subcutaneous injections are the standard for most self-administered medication. In addition, HCG solutions cannot be practically made from concentrate every few days.

Sublingual HCG

Dr. Belluscio, a well-known internist working in Argentina, was the first to demonstrate that oral HCG was at least 95% as effective as HCG by injection. His original report is available on his Internet site. Dr. Belluscio found significant weight loss compared with placebo as well as marked loss of fat around the abdomen and a general feeling of well-being with his oral HCG preparation.

Actually, there is no such thing as "oral" HCG. HCG cannot be swallowed. Like insulin, the normal stomach acids break down the HCG molecule to render it ineffective. Oral HCG really means taking it sublingually (under the tongue.) In the area right under everyone's tongue is a complex set of tiny capillaries which permit rapid absorption of drugs when placed there by an oral syringe. HCG taken sublingually is equally effective as HCG administered intramuscularly. The invention of oral HCG is good news for those who want to avoid injections.

Dosing HCG: Oral and Injection

If you are taking an HCG orally, you need to follow the directions of the manufacturer. In general, most prescription HCG preparations provide 250-500 IU twice a day. Many of the HCG preparations are prepared with bacteriostatic water, alcohol and vegetable glycerin to increase the absorption and keep the HCG stable. Most programs pro-vide 125-150 IU of HCG for injection once daily. In the table below, note that after 30 days the average weight loss did not differ whether taking the HCG by drops or injections.

Weight Loss: HCG Injection vs. Drops

	# of of dieters	% Weight Loss First 7 Days	% Weight Loss At 30 Days
HCG Drops	25	3.2%	10.1%
HCG Injections	28	4.1%	9.3%

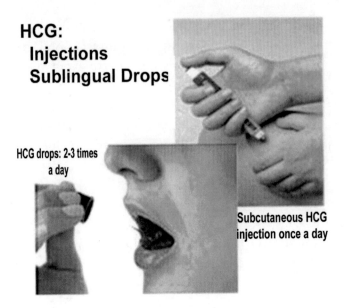

HCG:
Injections
Sublingual Drops

HCG drops: 2-3 times a day

Subcutaneous HCG injection once a day

Safety of Artificial Sweeteners:

Aspartame: Aspartame which is about 200 times sweeter than sugar was discovered in 1965 and used since 1981. It is unusual among nonnutritive sweeteners in that it is completely broken down during digestion into its basic components - the amino acids aspartic acid and phenylalanine plus a small amount of methanol. Aspartame was approved by the FDA for tabletop use in 1981 and for use in carbonated beverages in 1983. As of the early 2000s, the United States uses 75% of the aspartame produced in the world. Seventy percent of this amount is consumed in diet beverages. Aspartame is the nonnutritive sweetener that has received the greatest amount of negative attention in the mass media because of a study done in Europe in 2005 that linked aspartame to two types of cancer - leukemia, and lymphomas in female laboratory **rats**, (not humans).

In response to the 2005 European study, the National Cancer Institute (NCI) conducted a study of **half** a million people in the United States in 2006 and found no connection between cancer rates and aspartame consumption. The details of this study can be found in a fact sheet available on the NCI website. Another study conducted by the National Toxicology Program (NTP) of the National Institute of En-

vironmental Health Sciences (NIEHS) of aspartame as a possible car-
cinogen found **no** evidence that the sweetener causes cancer in humans. Aspartame is sold under the brand names NutraSweet, Equal,
and Sugar Twin (blue box).

Sucralose (Splenda): approved by the FDA in 1998, is unusual in that
it is the only nonnutritive sweetener made from sugar, but it is about
600 times as sweet as table sugar. Sucralose is manufactured from
sugar by substituting three chlorine atoms for three hydroxyl groups
in the sugar molecule. Only about 11 % of Sucralose is absorbed during digestion; the remainder is excreted unchanged. Sucralose is sold
under the trade name Splenda for table use.

Stevia: A traditional herb from a South American Plant

The Stevia plant is native to South and Central America but is also
cultivated in other areas such as Asia. It has a long history of culinary
and medicinal use with no known adverse effects. The leaves are reputed to be twice as sweet as table sugar. The sweet taste is attributed
to a synergistic effect of various compounds classified as rebaudio-
sides and steviosides which are reputed to be 200 times sweeter than
sugar. When the Stevia leaf is purified further a very potent sweetener is obtained called rebiana. Rebiana is now found on supermarket shelves incorporated into alternative sweeteners with sound-alike
names to Stevia, such as Truvia.

Truvia: a combination of Stevia and Erythritol

Truvía is a Stevia-based sugar substitute developed jointly by The
Coca-Cola Company and Cargill. It is distributed and marketed as a
tabletop sweetener as well as a food ingredient. Truvia is made of Rebiana, Erythritol, and natural flavors. Because it comes from the Stevia
plant, Cargill classifies it as a natural sweetener in addition to being a
non-nutritive sweetener. Since its launch in 2008, Truvia natural
sweetener has become the second best-selling sugar substitute in
unit s in the U.S. behind Splenda, surpassing Equal and Sweet'N Low.

Here are the position papers of the major academic institutions involved in the safety issue of artificial sweeteners:

"Available evidence suggests that consumption of aspartame by normal humans is safe and is not associated with serious adverse health effects." American Medical Association Council on Scientific Affairs report, published in The Journal of the American Medical Association, July 19, 1985

"Present levels of aspartame consumption appear to be safe for those who do not have PKU. . . . The blood phenylalanine levels reported in response to loading doses of aspartame in normal adults, and those heterozygous for the PKU gene do not seem to be sufficiently high to warrant concern of toxicity to the individual or even to a fetus during pregnancy." American Academy of Pediatrics Committee on Nutrition, Task Force on the Dietary Management of Metabolic Disorders, December 1985 Final Report.

"The American Diabetes Association finds the use of the two commercially available no caloric sweeteners saccharin and aspartame to be acceptable. The use of both sweeteners is encouraged for the particular advantages of each."

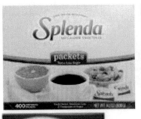
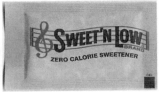
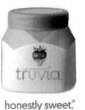
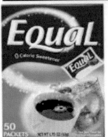
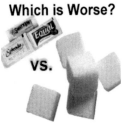
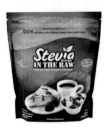

Which is Worse?

VS.

Phase 3: 1100 Calorie - High Metabolism

This phase begins right after you have completed phase 2, whether you do it for 10, 21 or even 42 days. You should have stopped the HCG two days before stopping the reduced calorie food plan. After that, you may begin the plan outlined in this chapter. Food selections, portions, and preparations are also illustrated with thumbnail pictures of food.

It is a weight loss plan based on keeping your metabolism working as fast as possible, avoiding hunger and losing weight. You can do this phase for 1-2 weeks and then return to phase 1 or 2, or you can do it for an indefinite time. It's easy and most of your favorite foods are here.

What to expect: A few carbs are added back as well as rye or whole wheat bread. Rice, pasta, potatoes, and sugars are still restricted. Most fruits are acceptable except for watermelon, the tropical fruits like bananas, mangos, pineapples, and all dried fruits such as figs, raisins, apricots, prunes, dates, and cranberries. Here are the limitations:

- **No sugar, dextrose, sucrose, honey, molasses, corn syrup, high fructose corn syrup**
- **No pasta, white rice, potatoes, yams, Limit bread to rye or whole wheat bread and at the most 2 slices a day or 1 low carb wrap or pitas. No cereal**
- **No food from fast food restaurants (except salads)**

When you see a chapter titled, "What's to Eat," you are probably expecting to find pages and pages of recipes, daily meal plans, and special foods that require shopping and cooking. You should eat what you like to eat and what you are accustomed to eating - only eliminating one or two of your problem foods and beverages. Keeping the food and beverage changes simple are the keys. If in doubt, calories and ease of portion control trump every other issue. Whether at home, in the school cafeteria, at sports games, or dancing lessons there are numerous good alternative foods and drinks that you will like.

Breakfast: Eat at Home, in the Car or at School, but Don't Skip It-Phase 3

Every weight loss study has found that both adults and children struggling with their weight are more successful if they have something to eat for breakfast. It's about metabolism and about control and making better choices later in the day. Protein is the key. For first 14 days, no cereal for breakfast. Rye, whole wheat or reduced carb bread is acceptable.

Secrets to a Good Breakfast- Phase 3

1. Drinking only juice is the same as skipping breakfast.
2. Skipping breakfast will lead to poor choices at lunch and loss of control over the foods for the rest of the day.
3. Convenience "rules" at breakfast - it's easy to avoid bagels, pastries, donuts, muffins, sugary cereals, and pop tarts if alternatives are easily available.
4. Choose foods high in protein, low in carbs with easy portion control.

What to Avoid at Breakfast Avoid having NO breakfast; also avoid only juice, bagels, muffins, sugary cereals, pancakes, donuts, pastries, fast foods. Avoid for first 14 days: cereal, white bread, rye or whole wheat bread is ok.

More about Breakfast Meal Menu

The breakfast menu above lists all the "free food and beverages". Two eggs count as one choice; one slice of whole wheat, rye, or whole grain toast counts as one choice, a high-protein shake counts as one or two choices, depending on the calories (total calories should be 190 or less).

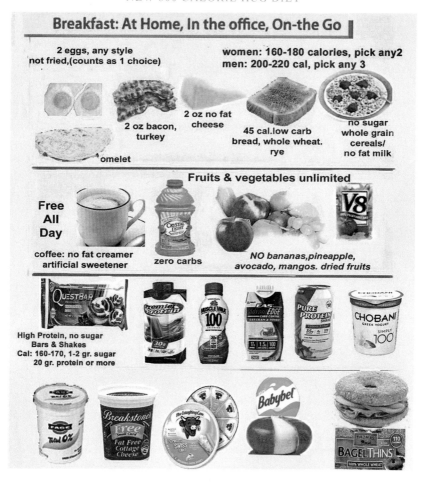

Breakfast: At Home, In the office, On-the Go

2 eggs, any style
not fried,(counts as 1 choice)

women: 160-180 calories, pick any 2
men: 200-220 cal, pick any 3

omelet

2 oz bacon,
turkey

2 oz no fat
cheese

45 cal.low carb
bread, whole wheat.
rye

no sugar
whole grain
cereals/
no fat milk

Fruits & vegetables unlimited

Free
All
Day

coffee: no fat creamer
artificial sweetener

zero carbs

NO bananas,pineapple,
avocado, mangos. dried fruits

High Protein, no sugar
Bars & Shakes
Cal: 160-170, 1-2 gr. sugar
20 gr. protein or more

Lunch: Small or Large Meal: Phase 3

Most people assume that their weight gain is due to snacking and making poor food choices or portion sizes at dinner. Although this ⁇ partly true, the mistakes made at lunch can far outweigh ⁇⁇ bad snacks or a large meal at dinner. Hard to believe?

Read on. A sandwich, sub, salad, or soup each average about 400 calories. Fast foods, fried foods, and hot dishes containing meat, chicken, rice, potatoes, or pasta (a large meal), typically average between 1,000 and 1,600 calories. The difference between the two types of meals -1200 cal.

Secrets to a Good Midday Meal: Keep it Small & Light & Eat Foods Served "Cold"

1. Few people that work inside a building all day can eat two large meals in a single day without gaining weight.

2. The time of day when a meal is consumed has no implication on weight gain or loss. Its better to save the large meal for the evening.
3. "Foods served cold" are low in calories & have easy portion control.
4. Eating a small lunch guarantees 1 large meal a day.
5. Sandwiches & wraps make great choices. They have easy, portion control, & high-calorie side dishes are seldom eaten with sandwiches or wraps. Hold the subs for a week or two.

What NOT to do at Lunch: Avoid skipping lunch, fast food, fried food, and meat, hot chicken, fish, pasta, rice, beans potatoes, pizza, or leftovers from the previous night's dinner. For the first 3 weeks limit the bread to whole wheat-2 slices per day.

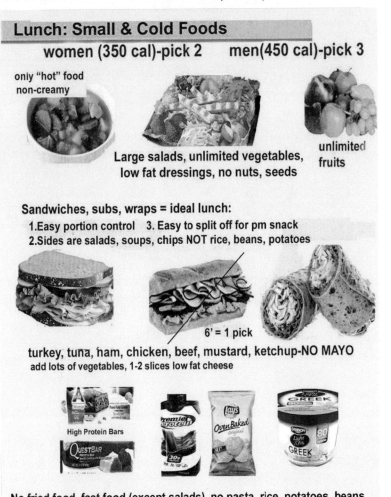

Lunch: Small & Cold Foods

women (350 cal)-pick 2   men(450 cal)-pick 3

only "hot" food
non-creamy

Large salads, unlimited vegetables, low fat dressings, no nuts, seeds

unlimited fruits

Sandwiches, subs, wraps = ideal lunch:
1.Easy portion control   3. Easy to split off for pm snack
2.Sides are salads, soups, chips NOT rice, beans, potatoes

6' = 1 pick

turkey, tuna, ham, chicken, beef, mustard, ketchup-NO MAYO
add lots of vegetables, 1-2 slices low fat cheese

High Protein Bars

No fried food, fast food (except salads), no pasta, rice, potatoes, beans
Limit bread to 2 slices whole wheat a day, limit sub for first 8 weeks

Dinner is the Big Meal of the Day: The Whole Family Eats Together Phase 3

Dinner is the large meal of the day. The family sits down together and has this meal together. It's an important time to talk about the day's events and future plans. Even 15-20 minutes set aside for this meal is better than nothing. The TV and homework are put aside. The protein and carb part of the dinner is where portion control counts. The biggest challenge to any meal of the day is fast food, because of its high-calorie content. In addition, foods with difficult portion control, such as proteins & carbohydrates, require special attention; the more caloric a food, the more critical its portion size. Below are suggestions for the dinner meal. Remember, portions are most important when eating beef, pork, and carbs. **For the first 2 weeks of this phase: eat anything you see in the picture below, but none of the carbs. After 2 weeks, you can return to Phase 1 and 2, or continue with this plan, watching portions and slowing resuming the carbs.**

Secrets to a Good Dinner: The Large Meal

1. Dinner should be the big meal of the day; it's time to relax and eat with the family.
2. Many items are completely or almost unlimited, including soups, salads, and vegetables served without butter or with low-fat or fat-free salad dressings.
3. Choose baked, barbequed, or grilled entrees, not fried dishes or fast foods.
4. Be careful with proteins and carbs that have portions that are difficult to control.

What NOT to do at Dinner

Avoid fast foods, fried foods, and large portions of meat, chicken. No pasta, potato, rice, or pizza yet.

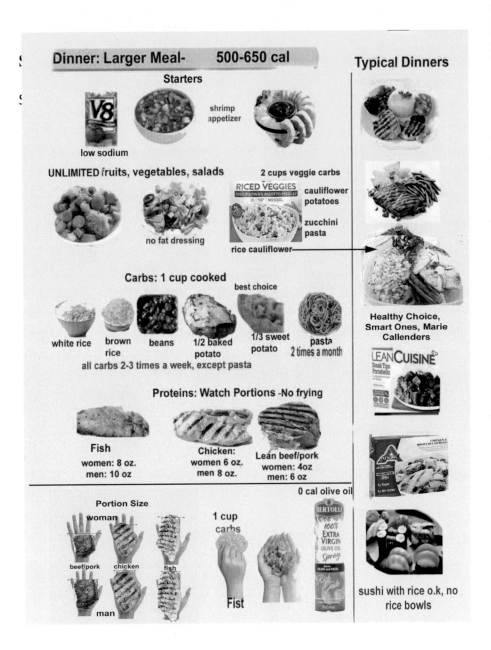

Dinner: Larger Meal-   500-650 cal

Starters

V8 low sodium

shrimp appetizer

UNLIMITED fruits, vegetables, salads

no fat dressing

RICED VEGGIES
CAULIFLOWER RISOTTO MEDLEY

rice cauliflower

2 cups veggie carbs

cauliflower
potatoes

zucchini
pasta

Carbs: 1 cup cooked

best choice

white rice   brown rice   beans   1/2 baked potato   1/3 sweet potato   pasta 2 times a month

all carbs 2-3 times a week, except pasta

Proteins: Watch Portions -No frying

Fish
women: 8 oz.
men: 10 oz

Chicken:
women 6 oz.
men 8 oz.

Lean beef/pork
women: 4oz
men: 6 oz

0 cal olive oil

Portion Size

woman

beef/pork   chicken   fish

man

1 cup carbs

BERTOLLI 100% EXTRA VIRGIN OLIVE OIL Spray

Fist

Typical Dinners

Healthy Choice,
Smart Ones, Marie
Callenders

LEANCUISINE

sushi with rice o.k, no
rice bowls

Snacks and desserts are useful. They will arm you with an option to prevent hunger and feelings of deprivation if they are the "right" snacks at the "right" times of the day. Here, is what you need to know about snacks - which ones to eat and which ones to avoid:

Secrets to Good Snacks: Phase 3

1. They provide protein, preventing falls in sugar in the afternoon.
2. They satisfy cravings, prevent hunger & feelings of deprivation.
3. Both convenience and cravings "rule." Seek 100-calorie snack bags of cookies, crackers, chips & 100 calorie portion controlled ice cream-like bars, light cheese, popcorn, low-fat yogurt, smoothies
4. The provide energy.

What Snacks to Avoid:

Traditional snack foods are high in calories, carbs, sugar, or fat, and often have serious portion control issues. They can easily exceed 300 or 400 calories. Avoid ice cream in cartons (low or not), cookies, candy, cake, chips, regular cheese, nuts, and seeds.

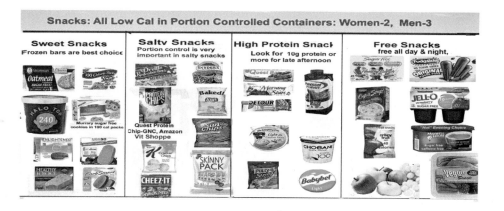

Books by Richard Lipman M.D.

The 100 Calorie Secret

New Pounds and Inches

La Dieta HCG

Restaurants and Recipes on HCG Diet

Diet Buddies: A Weight Loss Plan for Kids, Teens and Parents

The Qsymia Weight Loss Plan

Lose Weight with Belviq

Contrave, Belviq and Qsymia: Unlocking the Brain's Secret to Permanent Weight Loss

References

Dr. Simeons and HCG

Simeons, A.T. Pounds, and Inches, 1954

Simeons, A. T. The action of chorionic gonadotrophin in the obese. Lancet. 1954 (267):946-7

Simeons, A. T. Chorionic gonadotropin in the obese Lancet 1962 (279) No. 7219: 47-8. Santos, E.D., et al. In Vitro effects of Chorionic Gonadotropin on human adipose development J.Clin Endo. 2007(194) 313-325.

Simeons, A.T.W., Chorionic gonadotropins in geriatrics J. Am Geriat. Soc 1956;(36);4

Salans. L. P. et al, Human adipose tissue metabolism Am J Physiol 1968;(47): 153

Bellusico, Daniel, Utility of an Oral Presentation of HCG for the Management of Obesity: A Double-Blind Study 1994-2007 drbellusciomd@hcgobesity.org

Wolever, T.M., Jenkins, D.J. et al. The glycemic index: methodology and clinical implications Am J.Clin Nutr. 1991;(54): 846-854.

Astrup, A. The Satiety Power of Protein Am J Clin Nutr. 2005;(82):1-2

Rolls, B.J., Hetherington, M. et al. The specificity of satiety: the influence of foods of different macronutrient content on the development of satiety. Physiol Behav 1988;(43):145-53.

Asher, W.L., Harper, H. W., Effect of human Chorionic gonadotrophins on weight loss, hunger, and feeling of well being. Am J Clin Nutr. 1973 (26): 211-8.

FDA has published a notice that describes the safe levels of certain hormone-active ingredients that can be used in products. Other sources Include: The European Union, The US EPA research activities, The US EPA screening, and prioritization activities. FDA Statement about Parabens and estrogenic activity. FDA Statement about Phthalates and health effects.

Gusman, H. A. Chorionic gonadotropin in obesity. Further clinical observations. Am J Clin Nutr. 1969;(22); 686.

Lebon, P. Treatment of overweight patients with chorionic gonadotropins J Am Geriat Soc 1966;(14):116.

McGanity, W.J.Weight reduction—facts and fancy J Am Med Ass, 1962 (182): 1141.

LaPorte, D.J. Predicting attrition, and adherence to a very low- calorie diet. Int J Obes 1990; (14): 197-296

Sugar and Artificial Sweeteners

Jenkin D. J., Wolever, T. M. Glycemic index of foods: a physiological basis for carbohydrate exchange Am. J Clin Nutr. 1981; (34): 362-366.

Butchko, H.H., Stargel, W.W. Aspartamine: scientific evaluation in the post-marketing period. Reg Toxic Pharma. 2001;34: 221-33.

Drewnowski, A., Bellisle, F. Liquid calories, sugar, and body weight. Am J Clin Nutr. 2007;85(3): 651-61.

Drewnowski, A. Intense sweeteners and energy density of foods: implications for weight control. Eur J Clin Nutr. 1999; 53(10): 757-63.

Lean, M.E. J., Hankey, C. R. Aspartame and its effect on health. British Med Journal. 2004;329 :755-56.

American Dietetic Association (ADA). Position Statement on the Use of Nutritive and Nonnutritive Sweeteners Available online at:

http://www.eatright.org/cps/rde/xchg/ada/hs.xsl/home_3794_ENU_ HTML.htm.This position paper was adopted by the ADA's House of Delegates on October 18, 1992; reaffirmed on September 6, 1996; and reaffirmed again on June 22, 2000.

American Dietetic Association Position Paper: Use of Non nutritive and Nutritive Sweeteners J. Am.Diet.Ass 101(7) 2001L 810-9.

National Cancer Institute (NCI) Fact Sheet. Artificial Sweeteners and Cancer: Questions and Answers Bethesda, MD: NCI, 2006. Available online at

Http://www.cancer.gov/cancertopics/factsheet/Risk/artificial-sweeteners.

National Cancer Institute (NCI) Fact Sheet. Aspartame and Cancer: Questions and Answers Bethesda, MD: NCI, 2006.

Office of Food Additive Safety. Guidance for Industry: Frequently Asked Questions about GRAS College Park, MD: Office of Food Additive Safety, 2004.

Tordoff, M.G., Alleva, A. M. Effect of Drinking soda sweetened with aspartame or high-fructose corn syrup on food intake and body weight. Am J Clin Nutr. 1990;51: 963-9.

Vermunt, S. H. F., Pasman, W. J., et al. Effects of sugar intake on body weight: a review. Obesity Reviews. 2003; 4: 91-99.

Hunger Control in the HCG Diet = Success

Borzoei, S., Neovius, M., et al. A comparison of effects of fish and beef protein on satiety in normal weight men. Eur J Clin Nutr. 2006; 60(7): 897-902.

Cho, S., Dietrich, M., Brown, C. J. P., Clark, C. A., Block, G. The effect of breakfast type on daily energy intake and body mass index. J. Am Coll Nutr. 2003;22(4): 296-302.

Johnstone, A. M., Shannon, E., et al. Altering the temporal distribution of energy intake with isoenergetically dense foods given as snacks does not affect total daily energy intake in normal-weight men. Br J Nutr. 2000;83(1): 7-14.

Vander, Wal, J.S., Matin, J. M., et al. Short-term effect of eggs on satiety in overweight and obese subjects. J Am Coll Nutr. 2005;24(6):510-5.

Weigle D.S., Breen, P.A., Matthys, C.C., et al. A high-protein diet induces sustained reductions in appetite, ad libitum caloric intake, and body weight despite compensatory changes in diurnal plasma leptin and ghrelin concentrations. Am J Clin Nutr.1005;82: 41-8.

Farschchi, H. R., Taylor, M. A., Macdonald, I. A. Beneficial metabolic effects of regular meal frequency on dietary thermogenesis, insulin sensitivity and fasting lipid profiles in healthy obese women. Am J Clin Nutr. 2005;81: 16-24.

Is Exercise Needed on the HCG Diet?

Anderson, R., Wadden, T., Bartlett, S. J., Zemel, B., Verde, T. J., Franck-owiak, S. C. Effects of lifestyle activity vs. structured aerobic exercise in obese women. JAMA. 1999; 281(4): 335-40.

Ard, J. A. as quoted in "Cox, T.L., Malpede, C. Z., Desmond, R., A., Faulk, L. E., et al Physical activity patterns during weight maintenance following a low-energy density dietary intervention. Obesity. 2007; (15): 1226-32.

Carey, D. G., Nguyen T. V., et al. Genetic influences on central ab-dominal fat: a twin study. Int J Obes Relat Metab Disord. 1996; 20(8): 722-6.

Jakicic, J. M., Winters, C., Lang, W., et al. Effects of intermittent exer-cise and use of home exercise equipment on adherence, weight loss, and fitness in overweight women. JAMA. 1999; 282(16): 1554-60.

Malis, C., Rasmussen, E L., Poulsen, P., et al. Total and regional fat distribution is strongly influenced by genetic factors in young and elderly twins. Obes Res. 2005; 13(12): 2139-45.

Ravussin, R. Quoted in "Redman, L. M., Heilbronn, L.K., Martin, C.K., Alfonso, A., Smith, S, R., Ravussin, R. Effect of calorie restriction with or without exercise on body composition and fat distribution. A Ran-domized Trial. J. Clin Endocrinol Metab.2007;92(3): 865-72.

Saris, W. H. Exercise with or without dietary restriction and obesity treatment. Int J Obes Metab Disord. 1995; 19(Suppl 4): S113-6.

Stiegler, P., Cunliffe, A. The role of diet and exercise for the mainte-nance of fat-free mass and resting metabolic rate during weight loss.

Sports Med. 2006;36(3):239-62

Levine, J. A. Role of non-exercise activity thermogenesis in resistance to fat gain in humans. Science, 1999

Levine, J. A., Energy expenditure of non-exercise activity, Am. Soc Nutr. 2000.

McArdle, Katch & Katch, Exercise Physiology 5th ed, New York. Chapter 12: Diabetics Can Lose Weight Safely On HCG Plan

Wing, R.R. Blair, B., et al. Year-long weight loss treatment for obese patients with type II diabetes: Does including an intermittent very-low-calorie diet improve outcome? The American Journal of Medicine, Available online 17 June 2004.

Henry. R. R., et al, Benefits and limitations of very-low-calorie diet therapy in obese NIDDM. Diabetes Care, 1991.

Wing, R.R. VLCD and Weight Loss in Diabetics. Journal of the American Dietetic Association, 1995.

Wing, R.R., Marcus, M.D. Effects of a very-low-calorie diet on long-term glycemic control in obese type 2 diabetic subjects, Archives of Internal Medicine 1991

Alcohol and the HCG Diet.

Wang, L., et al Alcohol consumption, weight gain, and risk of becoming overweight in middle-aged and older women. Arch Intern Med. 2010 Mar 8;170(5):453-61.

French, M.D., Norton, E. C., et al. Alcohol consumption and body weight. Health Econ. 2010 Jul;19(7):814-32.

Sayen-Orea, C., et al, Type of alcoholic beverage and incidence of overweight/obesity in a Mediterranean cohort: The SUN project. Nutrition. 2010 Dec 9.

Cheers and Jeers for Alcohol.Consum Rep. 2011 Jan;76(1):10.

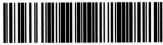

Made in the USA
Middletown, DE
06 May 2019